The Revolt A

"A truly outstanding contribution to critical work in this area. I simply loved reading the manuscript; by turns, questioning, thought-provoking, heart-breaking, challenging, yet always positive, sensitive to different outlooks, and with a real humanistic quality at its heart. I congratulate Professor Burstow and all the contributors to the book – the text is really moving, and made me (as a mental health academic) reflect upon a whole number of issues.... So inspiring!"
—Bruce Cohen, *Senior Lecturer in Sociology, University of Auckland, New Zealand*

"*Revolt against Psychiatry* is a celebration of living life on one's own terms. Defiant, relentless and radical, these anti/critical psychiatry dialogues extol activism and commitment from the edges of a world intent on not listening. A must-read for those thinking about the impact of institutional violence and what it means to be an expert through experience. A stellar contribution. Migwetch, everyone involved, and Mazel Tov."
—Jennifer Wemigwans, *Assistant Professor, OISE/University of Toronto, Canada, and author of* A Digital Bundle: Protecting Indigenous Knowledge Online

"A 'terrific read,' this latest book of Professor Bonnie Burstow's is an exceptional contribution to her already formidable repertoire. Consisting of 15 dialogical interviews with major players in the critical and antipsychiatry fields in different parts of the world, it is highly accessible, is enormously informative, and I predict will quickly become an indispensable go-to resource both for seasoned scholars and new students trying to wrap their mind around 'the revolt against psychiatry.'" *Venceremos*, Bonnie
—Stephen Ticktin, *member of the Medical Psychotherapy Association of Canada*

"In this amazing book, Bonnie Burstow gathers together a wide variety of expert global players in the critical/antipsychiatry movement. These stand-alone thought-provoking dialogues stimulate debate and offer a fascinating look into the opinions and strategies of people who challenge psychiatry. Passionate, gripping, heart-warming, and at times harrowing."
—Cheryl Prax, *survivor and member of the British activist group Speak Out Against Psychiatry, UK*

"Fantastic Work! Burstow's wide-ranging and deeply engaging series of dialogues not only exposes psychiatry as a pseudoscience but provides clues on how to resist and replace it. With a solid focus on human rights and an unwavering commitment to follow where the science leads, Burstow demonstrates that psychiatry isn't a service. It's a disservice."

—Irit Shrimrat, *co-founder of the Ontario Psychiatric Survivors' Alliance, Canada*

Bonnie Burstow

The Revolt Against Psychiatry

A Counterhegemonic Dialogue

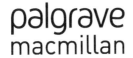

Bonnie Burstow
Ontario Institute for Studies in Education
Adult Education and Community Development
Toronto, ON, Canada

ISBN 978-3-030-23333-4   ISBN 978-3-030-23331-0   (eBook)
https://doi.org/10.1007/978-3-030-23331-0

© The Editor(s) (if applicable) and The Author(s), under exclusive licence to Springer
Nature Switzerland AG 2019
This work is subject to copyright. All rights are solely and exclusively licensed by the
Publisher, whether the whole or part of the material is concerned, specifically the rights of
translation, reprinting, reuse of illustrations, recitation, broadcasting, reproduction on
microfilms or in any other physical way, and transmission or information storage and retrieval,
electronic adaptation, computer software, or by similar or dissimilar methodology now
known or hereafter developed.
The use of general descriptive names, registered names, trademarks, service marks, etc. in this
publication does not imply, even in the absence of a specific statement, that such names are
exempt from the relevant protective laws and regulations and therefore free for general use.
The publisher, the authors and the editors are safe to assume that the advice and information
in this book are believed to be true and accurate at the date of publication. Neither the
publisher nor the authors or the editors give a warranty, express or implied, with respect to
the material contained herein or for any errors or omissions that may have been made. The
publisher remains neutral with regard to jurisdictional claims in published maps and institutional affiliations.

This Palgrave Macmillan imprint is published by the registered company Springer Nature
Switzerland AG
The registered company address is: Gewerbestrasse 11, 6330 Cham, Switzerland

This book is dedicated to Vern Harper—a psychiatric survivor and an Indigenous man, who, in his early years, was involuntarily psychiatrically incarcerated and, in the process, subjected to an insidious combination of racism and sanism. Now during his psychiatric incarceration Vern came perilously close to being electroshocked on two separate occasions—and who can say how his story would have unfolded had they actually gone through with the highly brain-damaging "procedure"? What happened? As the fates would have it, both times, when the moment when he was to be shocked arrived, the psychiatrist assigned him—a chap from India—unceremoniously entered the ECT room where Vern was lying and yanked the plug to the ECT machine out of the wall, exclaiming, "Not to my people, you don't!" (and no, the psychiatrist in question was not Indigenous). Now eventually Vern got himself out of the system and went on to live a singularly productive and worthwhile life in which he contributed substantially to society. A helper and a leader of people, whose brain—thank God!—had never been "fried", he went on to work at a huge number of social service agencies in Toronto. He became a highly respected and renowned elder, was known everywhere as the "urban elder"—the Toronto elder who could always be counted on to stand up for social justice. He co-organized the now legendary across-Canada trek to raise awareness of broken treaties (the Native People's Caravan). At the same time, he remained an outspoken member of the mad movement.

Late in his life, to the surprise of many of us, he started working at Centre for Addiction and Mental Health (CAMH), which is as mainstream psychiatry as you can get and where he served as in-house elder. Now while he had previously been involved in an early antipsychiatry publishing venture of mine—Shrink Resistant: The Struggle Against Psychiatry in Canada—*at this point, I lost touch with him, saddened by what appeared to be the movement's loss of him.*

Fast forward ten years—one day I heard that there had been a falling-out between Vern and CAMH—and I immediately had a message relayed to him, inviting him to phone me, which indeed he did. About 15 minutes into the phone call, I inquired about the falling-out and asked Vern what he had learned from his ten years' stretch working at CAMH. Without a moment's hesitation, he responded, "You know, Bonnie, if there is one thing that my ten years here has taught me, it is that what they do here, it is not good for my people." We schmoozed *for a while, and it was during this conversation I told him about this new dialogical book on which I was working. After telling me that he was eager to contribute once again to the movement in any way he could, he expressed a particularly keen interest in being interviewed for this very book, adding that in the interview, he would like to tell the story of almost being electroshocked for he felt that the story had the potential of doing good. All good. We never did get around to conducting the interview, however, for Vern was old and ill at this point; already he was beginning to fade; and before we were able to proceed further, he died.*

I tell Vern's ECT story here for besides that it fits, I promised him it would be in. Moreover, how Vern would have loved for this story to be the very first one told in this book, for what a model it provides! Would that more people would be saved by those around them taking "direct action"—for utterly unexpected though it was, that is precisely what happened here. Correspondingly, it is with profound respect that I dedicate this, my latest publication—The Revolt Against Psychiatry—*to the memory of psychiatric survivor, author, social service worker, Cree elder, medicine man, and activist Vern Harper. Old friend and ally,* Miigwetch!

Acknowledgments

First and foremost, I would like to acknowledge the contribution of all the people who entered into dialogue with me. Thank you Dr. Roland Chrisjohn, Dr. Peter Breggin, Robert Whitaker, Dr. Lauren Tenney, Kim Wichera, Dr. Ian Parker, Tatiana Castillo, Don Weitz, Nick Walker, Michael, Tina Minkowitz, Julie Wood, Dr. China Mills, and Oriel Varga. May the excellent work of all of you continue, and as years pass, may we all of us continue to reflect, rethink, and build together! Thanks too to everyone else who began the process for in your own way you also added to the knowledge. A special thanks to Margôt Smith for providing timely and thoughtful feedback on each of the chapters. Thank you Dr. Brenda LeFrançois, for your helpful recommendations along the way. Thank you graduate assistants, Oriel Varga, Nichole Schott, and Annalissa Crisostomo for your editing, feedback, and other assistance—and Oriel, how apt that we actually got to enter into dialogue together! Finally, thanks Palgrave Macmillan for agreeing to publish this book, and a special thanks to all editors that I have had the privilege to work with here, including but not limited to Rachel Daniel and Madison Allums.

CONTENTS

1 Introduction to This Book and to This Project   1

2 "It Is All About Racism": Dialogue with Indigenous Scholar and Activist Roland Chrisjohn   15

3 "Our Freedom of Speech Over Our Medical License": Dialogue with "The Conscience of Psychiatry"—Peter Breggin   33

4 Dialogue with Journalist Extraordinaire: Robert Whitaker   51

5 Dialogue with Survivor and Academic Lauren Tenney   69

6 On Berlin Runaway House: Dialogue with Wichera   83

7 Toward a Democratic Psychiatry? Dialogue with Ian Parker   93

8 "Activism Is My Real Job": The Mad Movement in Chile Dialogue with Tatiana Castillo   109

9 "There Is No Place on This Planet for Psychiatry Period!": Dialogue with Don Weitz   121

ix

X   CONTENTS

10   Autistic and Mad: Dialogue with Nick Walker   135

11   Dialogue with Indigenous Leader and Psych Survivor Michael   149

12   "This Is Not a Time to Lie Low": Dialogue with International Lawyer, Survivor, and Human Rights Advocate Tina Minkowitz   159

13   "I So Loved My Son that I Had to Promise Him that I'd Do Everything I Could": Dialogue with Mother and Archivist Julie Wood   175

14   Epistemicide: Dialogue with "Global Mental Health" Critic China Mills   191

15   "The Movement Is an Intrinsic Part of Who I Am": Dialogue with Bonnie Burstow   209

Epilogue   225

Appendices   233

Index   237

CHAPTER 1

Introduction to This Book and to This Project

While far from all books that touch on the topic of psychiatry (see, by way of contrast, Burstow 2015, Szasz 1970, Whitaker 2010), most books which invite us to think about psychiatry pose "onside" questions like: How do we treat the mentally ill? When do we use electroshock? And when are psychiatric drugs the better choice? Those are *hegemonic* books— books which accept the validity of psychiatry. This, by contrast, is a *counterhegemonic* book. It begins from what is more or less the opposite premises, has a very different purpose, and asks very different questions. What follows are some of those questions—to wit:

What pressures might we bring to bear to loosen the grip of psychiatry? We habitually seem to be losing the battle; so as thinkers, activists, radical practitioners, parents, and concerned members of society, how do we turn the situation around? What new challenges are we facing in organizing against psychiatry? How best might we contribute to a paradigm shift in what is erroneously known as "the mental health area"? How might we best articulate, describe, or explain a new and more promising paradigm? What models for prefigurative politics exist (you are engaging in the prefigurative when you incorporate into current practice aspects of the new society that you are trying to build)? What promising ventures are happening in different parts of the world? How might we bring together antipsychiatry with mad activism, with critical psychiatry, with critical disability, with radical neurodiversity? How do we counter the sexism, racism, and transphobia not only in psychiatry but in the movement(s) to counter

© The Author(s) 2019
B. Burstow, *The Revolt Against Psychiatry*,
https://doi.org/10.1007/978-3-030-23331-0_1

psychiatry? How might we understand the disagreement between the players in the movement itself? What does this fight actually mean to people? Of all the pressing social struggles in which they might become involved, exactly why did they end up taking on this one? And what keeps them involved year after year? Such are among the key questions addressed in this book.

As should be abundantly clear by this point, the general context in which this book is written is the reality of institutional psychiatry. As articulated in Burstow (2015, 2016), despite the high esteem in which it is held, and despite how unusual this claim may at the moment sound to you, psychiatry is a pseudo-medical profession; it is granted enormous power by the state; and it operates as a regime of ruling, in the process, as the United Nations (UN) itself has clarified (see Chap. 12), routinely infringing on people's human rights—all in the name of "help" and "protection". What adds insult to injury, despite the widespread societal belief in it, is the fact that it is a profession whose very foundational tenets have been repeatedly shown to be unscientific and lacking in validity, whose thinking is muddled, which is blatantly self-serving, and, moreover, whose "treatments" have been demonstrated again and again to do far more harm than good (see, in this regard, Burstow 2015, 2016; Breggin 1991, 2008; Healey 2012; Kirk and Kutchins 1992; Moncrieff 2008; Woolfolk 2001; Whitaker 2002, 2010; Whitaker and Cosgrove 2015; Szasz 1970; Foucault 1980). The very real injury done to vulnerable human beings is particularly alarming and is what unites the people featured in this book. Indeed, I suspect, every last one of us would nod in agreement with Robert Whitaker when he says, "The point is: I don't give a shit about psychiatry", that it is the individuals whose lives that they ravage that motivate him (see Chap. 4).

If the general context of the book is the harm wreaked by psychiatry itself, the book's focus is the people who challenge the institution. This book, to be clear, is first and foremost a book about a social justice movement and the counter-initiatives, counter-discourses, and individual journeys accompanying it. "Social movement" here is broadly defined so as to include anyone who is consciously part of what they see as a collective challenge to psychiatry, whether these be activists, theorists, teachers, researchers, parents, or radical practitioners. While inevitably such issues as the horror that is psychiatry is frequently touched on in the book, the primary focus is not the problems that psychiatry presents but the attempt to counter them. As the title suggests, it is about, rather, the "revolt against psychiatry".

Revolts, of course, are waged by real people. As such, what we witness in this book are not only strategies and counterstrategies—though these for sure are front and center—but also profoundly meaningful and highly personal journeys.

If the title of this book is key to what you find here, I would add, equally important is the subtitle—"A Counterhegemonic Dialogue". My project was to seek out major and otherwise important counterhegemonic theorists and players in the movement(s) and enter into dialogue with them. With care being taken to preserve the actual wording used verbatim, a shortened or abridged version of each of the dialogues that made it through the selection process subsequently became its own separate chapter in the book.

To give you a further sense of the process involved and the manuscript which emerged, what follows is an excerpt from the initial letter that I as interviewer and editor sent to prospective participants:

> I am writing to invite you to participate in an interview for an intended new book, whose provisional title is "The Revolt Against Psychiatry: In Dialogue with Bonnie Burstow". To be clear from the outset, I myself am 100 per cent antipsychiatry. You are being invited because you are an important figure in this conversation, and it is anticipated that readers will benefit from your words as well as from the exchange between us. As author/editor, I will be conducting the interviews and constructing the book. In the case of each chapter, a balance will be struck between trying to help the interviewee articulate their position, digging into/co-exploring together, focusing on unique meanings and unique paths, inviting reflection, and where the need arises, actively challenging, with the emphasis varying from chapter to chapter. The attempt is to both understand you in your uniqueness and at the same time enter into an engaged dialogue, even at times rethinking together. (Burstow, private correspondence, 2015)

While this was optional, interviewees were additionally given an opportunity to provide a written comment afterward either on the general topic or the dialogue itself and to include a list of their representative publications, which was subsequently included in the chapter. Correspondingly, at the end of the process each interviewee was given a copy of the edited down interview—now about a quarter of the original size—for their approval with slight corrections made as needed.

No hard or fast rules were used in deciding which part of the interview to use. General selection criteria, however, included:

1. The part sheds a particularly informative light on the interviewee themselves or on some aspect of either the revolt in general or the revolt in their part of the world.
2. Events of historical significance were being discussed and assessments made that might be useful in guiding future activism.
3. Light was cast on changes in the activist scene, what the new opportunities are, and what the special challenges are.
4. A formidable contribution to theory was being made.
5. Bottom lines were spelled out and activist principles were clarified.
6. Something original was being said or emerged.
7. Differences in perspectives were clarified.
8. In this section of the dialogue, something unexpected happened between interviewee and interviewer.

Significantly, two different, albeit related, understandings of dialogue underpin the invitation to participate and this book more generally. The first is existentialist Martin Buber's (1970), where dialogue is construed as an attempt to encounter the "other" and to understand the other in their particularity and, in turn, to be so encountered by them. A visual way of capturing the Buberian concept of dialogue is to imagine two people facing each other. The second understanding of dialogue is Paolo Freire's (1970), where dialogue is defined as an encounter between human beings mediated by the world in order to change the world. To encapsulate this second understanding, imagine two people not facing one another but jointly facing the world as they each go about world-changing praxis. The beauty of investing this book in dialogue in general, and these specific approaches to dialogue in particular is not only are a range of people drawn out, but there are spirited disagreements. Everyone's experiences and engagements with the world enter in. Correspondingly, there are magical moments where insight is reached that could not be achieved individually. In the "back-and-forth" between people in dialogue—that is, where much of the magic happens.

Albeit they are "distant relatives" only, there is some similarity between this book and two earlier ones. The first is an anthology of writings by Canadian mad studies theorists (see LeFrançois et al. 2013). The difference—and it is huge—is that the earlier book is not a book of dialogues, and it is focused solely on Canada. The second—called *Szasz Under Fire* (Schaler 2004), indeed, has a dialogical aspect to it. It is composed of written critiques of the writings of legendary critical psychiatry theorist

1 INTRODUCTION TO THIS BOOK AND TO THIS PROJECT 5

Thomas Szasz, plus Szasz's written responses to each of the critiques. The differences are—and once again they are enormous—that the understanding of dialogue in the Szasz book is strictly confrontational; these are written critiques—not face-to-face oral conversations—and the focus is on Szasz as opposed to being on-the-world; there is no attempt whatever to encounter, to co-imagine, or to create together; and theory—not activism—is central. In short, while there is some resemblance to earlier literature, this book is unique, and it is largely the dialogical nature of this book that makes it so.

What adds further to this book's distinctness and importance is that unlike with other books in the area, the single biggest focus is on the question of psychiatry abolition. Indeed, herein lies a critical part of the book's challenge. In this regard, while some of the interviewees are avowed abolitionists (e.g., Tenney and Weitz), whereas others are reformers who either reject or at least are wary of the abolitionist position (e.g., Mills and Whitaker), all interviewees are in dialogue with me—an abolitionist—and in all cases, I invite the interviewee to wrestle precisely with the question of psychiatry abolition. What is their position on this utterly vital question? Why do they take this position? Do they in any way want to qualify their position? As such, the issue of abolition per se is uniquely central to this book.

For whom is *The Revolt Against Psychiatry* written? People who are part of the struggle against psychiatry. People critical of psychiatry who want to learn more about the revolt against it, perhaps with the thought of actively joining, perhaps out of simple curiosity. People who just may end up hearing from friends that there is something in this book that they should think of checking out—perhaps concerned parents, perhaps lawyers. Activists and scholars interested in social movement theory, especially those with a passion for bringing together theory and practice. People intrigued by or who intrinsically value dialogue. People keen on fathoming the personal behind the political. Social scientists. Students of all types.

And what can you as reader expect to get out of the book? An introduction to key players in the area —what they think and do, how they ended up where they are. A sense of the variety of the people involved and the differences between them Insight into how personal/political transformation happens. A window onto activism in the current era. An overview of the struggle against psychiatry in different parts of the world. An introduction to key debates in the field. Ideas about what you yourself or your group might do. Insight into how people find themselves in the process of finding their social justice calling.

6   B. BURSTOW

Now you may be thinking that this book is not exactly aimed at the general public. And for sure that is true *to a point*. And if you regard yourself more or less as a typical member of the general public, that reality in itself may tempt you to put the book down. My invitation is to reserve judgment and dip into it anyway for the general public was very much on my mind when constructing this book. Indeed, to an appreciable degree, you are the intended audience. Besides that, there are thought-provoking conversations, and besides that, much of this book is a truly fascinating "read"; we are in an emergency right now, and as a dweller on this planet, you direly need to know about it. How else are you going to contribute to the healing or even the safeguarding of the world? Correspondingly, as you delve further and further into the book, as you take in such horrors as that there has been a 35-fold increase in the number of children given psychiatric diagnoses in recent years, as you come face to face with the plight of a mother whose child's "suicide" can be traced to the "psychiatric treatment", and it dawns on you how easily that could be you and your child, as you come to terms with the fact that mad Black men who have done no one any harm are being shot by police at astronomical rates, as you see just how pervasively the Global South is being colonized by the Global North with local practices both dismissed and co-opted, as you fathom how routine and extensive the manipulation and misrepresentation of psychopharmaceutical research is, as you begin to see the pivotal role of psychiatry in genocide, as you truly let yourself grapple with Lauren Tenney's haunting but, alas, realistic prognosis (see Chap. 5)—that if things go on as they are now, 60 years hence there may not be a single person alive who actually knows what it is like not to have a psychiatric diagnosis—you are likely to understand the urgency. Correspondingly, as you find yourself facing the urgency, this book may start to feel utterly indispensable to you—for the dialogues within hold clues as to what you might do about the situation.

Interviews with 14 key figures, in total, are included. While not all psychiatric survivors so identify, I am pleased to report that almost half the people featured are survivors. Correspondingly, half are women. Interviewees include activists, practitioners, mad folk, artists, and scholars. With my commitment being not only to showcase "the usual suspects"—albeit many of these are included—but every bit as importantly to capture and honor diversity: Two of the interviewees are Indigenous; five are Jews (with some of Jewish interviewees identifying as of color and others as white); two are trans; many are multiracial; and several are BIPoC. What is significant here—from early on in this project, I was driven by an unshakeable commitment not to stop looking and interviewing until the book included at least two Indigenous chapters, each with a powerful analysis. By the same token, I was committed to ensuring that people of color were represented, as were issues of colonialism. A balance, to be clear, was struck between including acknowledged leaders and achieving diversity. The inevitable upshot is that while some absolutely wonderful leaders are not included, a goodly number are; additionally, several comparatively new but immensely powerful voices are also heard. Correspondingly, in the interest of honoring diversity, instead of beginning the book with a chapter on what is commonly (and erroneously) thought of as "general resistance", I began with a markedly Indigenous chapter—as it happens, an absolutely brilliant one. Figuring likewise is a variety of different movement affiliations, political perspectives, and regions.

While commonly combining several of these, the allegiances of the dialoguers featured here range between antipsychiatry, critical psychiatry, the mad movement, the disability rights movement, and the neurodiversity movement (for a quick introduction to the nature of each of the movements and for help grasping the distinctions between them—the reader is referred to Appendix A). While most of the dialoguers are left wing, one is manifestly on the right, and one identifies as neither right nor left. Correspondingly, countries represented in a meaningful way include not only Canada and the US (which for sure are paramount) but also Germany, the UK, Chile, and India.

The themes that have emerged are far too numerous to name. To identify some absolutely pivotal ones, however, major themes include abolition versus reform; the problem of co-optation; activism; the use of language; coming to critical awareness; creating a new paradigm; direct action; engagement with the left; racism and antiracism; genocide; the ever-growing danger to youth worldwide; The Convention on the Rights of Persons with Disabilities (CRPD); the North—South divide; the colonial travesty that is the "Movement for Global Mental Health"; feminism; Marxism; anarchism; libertarian; establishing a grassroots press; creating participant led alternatives; making the movement truly international; being a different type of practitioner; teaching as activism; bringing survivors and radical professionals together; and building a better world. Particularly recurring and pivotal is how to work around media bias by, in essence, becoming one's own press (e.g., Breggin, Chap. 3; Whitaker, Chap. 4; Tenney, Chap. 5; and Wood, Chap. 13). On a deeper level, pivotal, likewise, are coming to awareness, and finding the core of who one is in the process of becoming more political (e.g., Weitz, Chap. 9; Michael, Chap. 11; and Burstow, Chap. 15). Which brings us to the chapter-by-chapter breakdown, beginning with the first of the dialogues (Chap. 2):

Chapter 2—"It's All About Racism: Dialogue with Indigenous Scholar and Activist Roland Chrisjohn"—is at once a scrupulously honest and politically astute piece. In it, we are introduced to an Indigenous activist and scholar, who, upon witnessing the suicide of one of his people, became a psychologist ("I was as big an idiot as anybody", acknowledges Roland), then moved on to become a leading critic of the psy disciplines. Drawing on no less formidable a philosopher than Ludwig Wittgenstein, Roland astutely points out that the psy disciplines proceed as if the empirical were capable of providing conceptual clarity—when that is exactly what empirical investigation *cannot* do. He demonstrates systematically the decimation of Indigenous culture. And he declares the psychiatrization of Indigenous people a "continuation of genocide". Drawing on Marxism, anarchism, and Indigenous culture, correspondingly, he masterfully points out that whatever else Indigenous people were, "we weren't capitalists". His repeated use of the Holocaust to show the absurdity of the pathologizing approach to the problems facing Indigenous communities is particularly thrilling. The sheer brilliance and radical thrust of this piece cannot be overstated. In short—Roland "rocks".

Likewise, brilliant and highly principled is the figure featured in Chap. 3, "Our Freedom of Speech Over Our Medical License: Dialogue with the 'Conscience of Psychiatry' Peter Breggin". A radical psychiatrist and researcher who quickly came to see through the folly of his own profession, Peter shares several of his own strategies for combating psychiatry: From issuing medical alerts; to establishing an honorary blogger site; to creating a training program for a new, nutrition-aware, and loving kind of counsellor. He also elaborates on his own right-wing politics and how it came about. If you have a formulaic politic which identifies us lefties only as allies and the right-right wing as problematic, besides reading Peter's other publications—for Peter is an undisputed leader—you owe it to yourself to read this eye-opening chapter. You won't be disappointed.

In Chap. 4—"Dialogue with Journalist Extraordinaire: Robert Whitaker"—we are afforded an insider glimpse into the co-optation of the media and how to counter what is happening by creating one's own media. Robert walks us through the development of the world's most popular critical psychiatry Internet site—*Mad in America*. Correspondingly, after a spirited back-and-forth between interviewee and interviewer, we receive the following gutsy acknowledgment from the figure who is arguably the world's leading advocate of psychiatric reform: "Put this down to my own person opinion only, okay? Do I think psychiatry is reformable? No, not in a big picture way."

Are you interested in participatory research as resistance? In blog radio? Do you want to gain insight into the special challenges faced by antipsychiatry activists today? Has it dawned on you that some of the current critical psychiatry spaces may not, in fact, be movement spaces? Are you worried about what the future will look like as psychiatry continues to grow by leaps and bounds? Then take a deep breath and proceed to Chap. 5, "Dialogue with Survivor and Academic Lauren Tenney".

Chapter 6, "On Berlin Runaway House: Dialogue with Kim Wichera", provides a window onto antipsychiatry in Germany. What is equally important, it showcases a highly promising "alternative" to psychiatry—a house where people can go to recover from psychiatry—one, moreover, which has long served as a model because of the scrupulousness of the emphasis on choice, self-direction, and mutual support. Correspondingly, in this chapter, we discover that in Germany, the left and the feminist movements are strongly allied with antipsychiatry.

Chapter 7, "'Toward a Democratic Psychiatry?': Dialogue with Ian Parker", features a critique of the psy complex from the left, with a critical distinction made by Ian between slavishly following "moral" rules and actually being ethical. The resistance scene in Great Britain is discussed, in particular, the initiatives associated with the magazine *Asylum*. While there is sizable agreement between interviewer and interviewee overall, there are also moments of profound difference. To whet your appetite by quoting from one such exchange, this with respect to the use of words, "Are you saying it's not possible to reclaim?" asks Ian incredulously. "It's possible to reclaim the word 'asylum'", I answer, "but no, it is not possible to reclaim the word 'psychiatry'."

An incredible change is sweeping over Chile. Over the past half-decade, a vibrant mad movement has emerged, one so radical that it smacks of anarchism. "We don't just want to change the 'mental health system", states Chilean activist Tatiana Castillo. "We are out to change society." Consciousness-raising is happening both in and outside of academic spaces, in the vast majority of the cases, with mad people as opposed to professional allies assuming center stage. Houses to retreat to, mad women's c.r. groups, bringing together mad activists and their allies from across

Latin America all figure in what is happening. For a window onto these exciting new developments, see Chap 8: "Activism Is My Real Job: The Mad Movement in Chile: Dialogue with Tatiana Castillo".

In Chap. 9 ("There Is No Place on This Planet for Psychiatry—Period": Dialogue with Don Weitz), readers are treated to two antipsychiatry veterans—Don Weitz and me—evaluating our decades of activism together as well as musing over directions for the future. Focal topics include decent survivor-centered alternatives, human rights violations, abolishing electro-convulsive (ECT), and the need to bring back direct action. Don also shares a revealing part of his own personal history—how he went from being a "psychiatric patient", to being a "mental health" professional, to being a psychiatric survivor/antipsychiatry activist. Speaking of "gutsy" personal transformation!

In Chap. 10: "Autistic and Mad: Dialogue with Nick Walker", survivor and neurodiversity theorist Nick Walker articulates the difference between "the neurodiversity paradigm" and the "medical paradigm". Highlights include the discussion of Nick's publishing ventures, the introduction of the concept "cognitive liberty", and Nick's vision of how to go about creating a better world. "I'm not in a fight", announces Nick triumphantly. "I'm building something."

The next of the dialogues was supposed to have been with Black scholar Idil Abdillahi, the principal focus being the conflation of mad, Black, and dangerous and the concomitant ongoing fatal police shooting of Black mad men in Canada. While, unfortunately, unforeseen circumstances prevented this, I would nonetheless invite you to learn about this area. I would draw your attention, for example, to the shooting of mad Black man Abdirahman Abdi in Ottawa (see https://ottawacitizen.com/news/local-news/timeline-everything-we-know-in-the-abdirahman-abdi-case) and, similarly, the Toronto police's killing of Andrew Loku (https://ottawacitizen.com/news/local-news/timeline-everything-we-know-in-the-abdirahman-abdi-case). Correspondingly, do consider reading Idil's excellent article on anti-Black sanism (Meeria et al. 2016).

Adding to the theme of racism generally and racism against Indigenous people in particular, Chap. 11 (Dialogue with Indigenous Leader and Psych Survivor Michael) ushers us into the horror that was the Sixties Scoop (where Indigenous infants were stolen from Canada and Mexico and adopted out to white parents in the US), with a further look at the psychiatrization, that, alas, all too often followed. Michael recounts the horrendous story of his being abducted as a child himself, deprived of his heritage, and later twice psychiatrized. "Would they do this to white people?" Michael pointedly asks. One highlight of the chapter is the healing that eventually came to Michael when he partook of Indigenous ceremony. The chapter ends with Michael reflecting on the possibility of Indigenous psychiatric survivors joining the antipsychiatry movement and the two creating testimony together.

In Chap. 12 ("This is Not a Time to Lie Low"), we make the acquaintance of the international human rights lawyer and activist Tina Minkowitz. Clarifying what is mandated by the UN's Convention on the Rights of Persons with Disabilities (CRPD) and explaining its significance for psychiatric survivors, Tina introduces readers to such groundbreaking developments as a presumption of capacity that is actually "irrebuttable". She speaks of recognizing and grabbing the moment at a time when others were intent on "lying low". In this eye-opening chapter, Tina walks us through not only the strengths of the CRPD but also the ways in which it is currently being watered down, sidelined, and co-opted. Correspondingly, she signals the fights that lie ahead.

Are you a parent who has begun to suspect that your child is being harmed by psychiatry? Are you suspicious about what psych drugs actually do? Are you itching for tips on how to get good information about the psych drugs out into the world? If so, take a look at Chap. 13 (Dialogue with Mother and Archivist Julie Wood). In this moving and eye-opening dialogue, you will encounter the heart-wrenching tale of a mother who lost her son to psychiatric drugs. Correspondingly, you will witness her transformation into a critic, an archivist, and an activist. Other highlights of this chapter include an introduction to a website which contains accurate information about the psychiatric drugs and a thought-provoking conversation on why and how parents might become a leading critical/antipsychiatry force in their own right.

Chapter 14 ("Epistemicide": Dialogue with China Mills) takes us onto the world stage, exploring, in particular, the North—South divide and the colonization, racism, and empire-building involved. It is the most dialogical of the chapters, with China and I "*schmoozing*" together on key debates within the movement. Focal are a strong analysis of the colonialism at the core of the "Movement for Global Mental Health", the value of pluralism, a reassuring glimpse into the integration of feminism in the survivor movement in India, the prioritizing of local grassroots approaches to healing. Additionally, in an attempt to shed light on one of the growing tensions within the movement and to find a constructive way forward, the two of us endeavor to wrap our minds around the thorny question of what and what is not appropriation. Thank you once again, China.

Finally, in what is a turnabout, the person interviewed in Chap. 15—"The Movement is an Integral Part of Who I Am"—is me, Dr. Bonnie Burstow. Having walked the reader through how it is I became an antipsychiatry activist, I shed light on such topics as what constitutes good strategic activism, what mistakes we have made as activists, what the take-away lessons are, the attrition model of psychiatry abolition, and the use of the arts in activism. What is particularly unique about this dialogue is that both teaching per se and being a counterhegemonic trauma practitioner emerge as forms of antipsychiatry activism in their own right.

And with this turnabout, the manuscript itself starts drawing to a close. Though not without an epilogue first that drives home where we have been, its relevance—and, yes, of course, where we might "go with it".

Such then is the book and such are the reasons for it. These are the people that you will encounter. These are examples of the issues, thoughts, interactions, and conversations that you will witness, though, more to the point, that you will find yourself smack in the middle of!

Correspondingly, these are the journeys that lie ahead.

REFERENCES

Breggin, P. (1991). *Toxic psychiatry: How therapy, empathy, and love must replace the drugs, electroshock, and biomedical theories of the "New Psychiatry".* New York: St. Martin's Press.

Breggin, P. (2008). *Brain-disabling treatments in psychiatry: Drugs, electroshock, and the psychopharmaceutical complex.* New York: Springer.

Buber, M. (1970). *I and thou* (W. Kaufmann, Trans.). New York: Charles Scribner's Sons.

Burstow, B. (2015). *Psychiatry and the business of madness: An ethical and epistemological accounting.* New York: Palgrave Macmillan.

Burstow, B. (2016). *Psychiatry interrogated: An institutional ethnography anthology.* New York: Palgrave Macmillan.

Foucault, M. (1980). *Power/Knowledge* (C. Gordon, Trans.). New York: Pantheon.

Freire, P. (1970). *Pedagogy of the oppressed.* New York: Continuum International Publishing Group.

Healey, D. (2012). *Pharmageddon.* Berkeley: University of California Press.

Kirk, S., & Kutchins, H. (1992). *The selling of the DSM: The rhetoric of science in psychiatry.* New Brunswick: Transaction Publishers.

LeFrançois, B., Menzies, R., & Reaume, G. (Eds.). (2013). *Mad matters: A critical reader in mad studies*. Toronto: Canadian Scholars' Press.

Meeria, S., Abdillahi, I., & Poole, J. (2016). An introduction to anti-Black sanism. *Intersectionalities, 5*(3), 18–35.

Moncrieff, J. (2008). *The myth of the chemical cure: A critique of psychiatric drug treatment*. London: Palgrave Macmillan.

Schaler, J. (Ed.). (2004). *Szasz under fire: A psychiatric abolitionist faces his critics*. New York: Open Court Publishing.

Szasz, T. (1970). *The manufacture of madness*. New York: Harper and Row.

Whitaker, R. (2002). *Mad in America: Bad science, bad medicine and the enduring mistreatment of the mentally ill*. New York: Perseus Books.

Whitaker, R. (2010). *Anatomy of an epidemic: Magic bullets, psychiatric drugs, and the astonishing rise of mental illness in America*. New York: Broadway Paperbacks.

Whitaker, R., & Cosgrove, L. (2015). *Psychiatry under the influence: Institutional corruption, social injury, and prescriptions for reform*. New York: Palgrave.

Woolfolk, R. (2001). The concept of mental illness. *The Journal of Mind and Behavior, 22*, 151–187.

CHAPTER 2

"It Is All About Racism": Dialogue with Indigenous Scholar and Activist Roland Chrisjohn

Roland Chrisjohn is a long-time Indigenous scholar and activist, a member of the Onyota'a:ka (Oneida Nation, part of the Iroquois Confederacy or League of Haudenosaunee), and a Professor of Native Studies at St. Thomas University, which itself is located on Canada's east coast. He is known, among other things, for stating unequivocally that the psychiatrization of Indigenous people is part of genocide.

I came across Roland only a short time ago for his voice and work are not typically included in critical or antipsychiatry theorizing. A serious omission, that it behooves us to correct. For far too long, let me add, this movement has been largely settler and white.

BB: I can't tell you how delighted I am to have the opportunity to interview you!

RC: Really? Why?

BB: That's easy, Roland. Because you are a brilliant Indigenous scholar who is into Indigenous resurgence and who has a profound critique of psychiatry. I can't for the life of me figure out why I didn't discover you twenty years ago

RC: Well, I discovered you *more than* twenty years ago. I used to teach out of your book *Radical Feminist Therapy* [Burstow 1992].

BB: Good to know. Anyway, I couldn't imagine doing a book of this sort this without a powerful Indigenous voice included. And on this issue, this was not easy to find. While I am in no way implying

© The Author(s) 2019

B. Burstow, *The Revolt Against Psychiatry*,

https://doi.org/10.1007/978-3-030-23331-0_2

16   B. BURSTOW

that a critique of psychiatry is missing among Indigenous people, a problem that I faced when I contacted Indigenous scholars to see if they would take part in this project, while using words like "over-representation", most wanted an alliance of some sort with psychiatry, and many would make statements like, "My people need the medications."

RC: (groan)

BB: So to varying degrees, despite the existence of meaningful critique, I was hearing from people who were buying into the standard psychiatric line, whereas I see the psychiatrization of Indigenous people as part and parcel of colonization.

RC: I would go further and say "genocide".

BB: Genocide, unquestionably. First children were stolen from their parents—and blatantly, that was genocidal—and then when parents complained, they were labeled insane and institutionalized by psychiatry.

RC: Precisely.

BB: So let me ask you something personal. Given the hugely problematic nature of the psy professions, way back when, as a young Indigenous person and indeed an activist, how did you come to go into psychology?

RC: A friend of mine committed suicide. We had just started a chapter of American Indian Movement in Canada—this was 1972. We wanted to take back our reserve, which had been taken from our grandfathers' generation and turned over to white farmers. Our grandfathers were dispossessed. And our fathers followed their fathers. They didn't take up farming again. And our generation said: There is all this farming equipment, and there is all this land that the white farmers don't want any more. Why don't we plow it? Anyway, we gathered together a group of people and put much of the acreage under cultivation. Now, one day a member of our group killed himself. I had majored in psychology at university, and I'm sitting there thinking: I'm supposed to know something about people having problems. And it never occurred to me that one of my best friends was suicidal. So I said, however much I think I know about the subject, it's not enough. What I need to do is go back and get a degree in psychology.

BB: I can surely understand how that happened. And did you think at the time that psychology was a benign discipline that would be of help to your people?

RC: Indeed, I did. I was as big an idiot as anybody.

BB: (laughter) I am always surprised at hearing about all these radical people going into psychology, especially people whose communities have been so badly oppressed.

RC: You know, I don't think it's accidental. Of course, once you get in there, you realize that psychology isn't self-critical. The problem is that you end up "buying" the standard line because you don't hear anything else.

BB: Yes, and all the language is vested in this individualized way of thinking.

RC: And not only that, there is all this status and power associated with the field.

BB: Eventually you must have found yourself at odds with your colleagues in psychology who mainly were not very critical. How did that change come about?

RC: I was studying under someone who was slightly critical. He said that psychology wasn't philosophically deep enough and that it had to be pushed to its limit; and he was developing methodologies for that. I learnt statistics and multivariate analysis, but at the same time, I kept pushing on the philosophical end because I concluded that my mentor himself was not philosophical enough. When I began teaching at university, I went deeper into the mathematics, and around 1984, there came a moment when I said, "This can't work. This is entirely wrong. And if this is entirely wrong, what is entirely right?"

BB: How did this happen?

RC: I picked up a copy of Baker's and Hacker's first volume of their analysis of Wittgenstein's *Philosophical Investigations* [see Baker and Hacker 1980/2014] and suddenly I realized that in this very book lie the philosophy needed to overturn psychological thinking to overturn it in its entirety. What it shows is that psychological thinking is "dead in the water". You know, there is a reason why Wittgenstein is marginalized. If we take him seriously—and I think we have to—then everything psychology and psychiatry does is wrong. Now I had already heard of Thomas Szasz. And in fact, we were friends.

BB: Szasz was brilliant.

RC: A right winger but brilliant. Now he made some hints in the direction of Wittgenstein.

BB: Let's zero in on this. What aspect of Wittgenstein were you focusing on? What is it that announced and still announces to you that the psych disciplines must be set aside?

RC: (laughter) Very simply: his explaining that conceptual clarification is not an empirical task.

BB: (laughter) And that's exactly right.

RC: The point is that the psy disciplines treat the empirical as if it could provide conceptual clarity. As then you can build the scales upward. Now what I had run into mathematically is a phenomenon call Simpson's Paradox [for details, see https://en.wikipedia.org/wiki/Simpson%27s_paradox]. It's a technical matter. And what it means is that with any relation, you can always disaggregate it. So think of it this way: Here's IQ and school achievement, okay? You have a diagram showing IQ scores and school achievement scores. Now with any diagram, you are going to be able to say: Let me break this down a little bit further. You might say, for example, "let me look at the boys and the girls." Or "let me look at different minority groups." Simpson found in 1951 that unless it's a perfect functional relation—and there are none mathematically in the "social sciences"—then you are always going to be able to disaggregate in such a way that either the relationship goes away entirely or it reverses itself. So here's the problem: How do you build a system about which you can say "I know that it works"? When what you have to say instead is that at some level of disaggregation, I know that it *doesn't* work.

BB: Correct.

RC: So psychology has locked itself into this false idea for a very long time. And they still have no idea what they're talking about. And they keep thinking that they are going to gather data and it will solve everything. Take PTSD, something that you yourself critique. They operate under the premise that sooner or later, we are going to gather enough data to understand it.

BB: When it's an invented concept in the first place.

RC: Exactly.

BB: You can't say, what's going to give substance to my generalization when the generalization is arbitrary and you are making it for political reasons.

RC: Yup. And the social sciences—psychology, psychiatry, all start from the premise: We are scientists; and therefore, if we gather enough data, we will figure everything out. But as Wittgenstein so brilliantly argued, conceptual clarification is logically prior to the empirical investigation. What follows, if you want to achieve conceptual clarification, it is pointless to proceed empirically.

BB: Very interesting. And the ramifications are huge. So this underpins your overall critique of psychiatry, regardless of who is being psychiatrized?

RC: Yes.

BB: A solid and fundamental critique. If we could focus in now explicitly on Indigenous people and the psych disciplines, how would you summarize what has happened here?

RC: Psychology has depoliticized what is essentially a political issue; it has pathologized people who are not sick; you know, it is all about racism. I am working on a book on racism, and I have to look at how Canada developed its policies. Genocide is a Canadian policy. They call it "assimilation" and then pretend that they don't practice assimilation, but we are talking about genocide. The point is that they wanted to vacate Native title; and they were not allowed to kill us. Now the US had the same issue at the end of the war of 1812. They didn't have title to the US. The crown likewise did not have title to Canada. And so when you want the land, how are you going to deal with this situation? Pathologization is key to the answer. The institutionalization of the pathology of Native people happened on both sides of the border simultaneously. The question they asked themselves was: Can savages be civilized or are they incorrigible? In the United States, they decided that savages were mostly incorrigible and therefore the settlers were entitled to kill the savages, with the understanding that those ones that they could salvage, they would. In Canada, by contrast, the British North America Act did not allow them to slaughter us. Moreover, we were allies—we saved Canada's ass twice. So all they could do is embark on the project of turning us into something "useful" or letting us die. That was the policy. Canada's reasoning was: The US has assured us that the Aboriginal population is dying out, so why not help Nature on its way? So, for example, we won't spend money on tuberculosis—because that's a racial problem. And so on. And Indians did die from such disorders. But the causes were always attributed to the existence of inherent racial insufficiencies.

BB: The overt psychiatrization of Indigenous people proceeded with similar rationales given. The justification for the psychiatric treatment is that there is something inherently wrong in the blood, in the lineage, whatever. Similar when it came to what education would be provided.

RC: Precisely. You know, they literally said, when it comes to Indians, the left side of their brain does not work. What does that mean? Well, in Saskatchewan it meant, we shouldn't have them take math classes or logic classes or learn grammar. Rather, we'll show them how a broom works and things like that. This whole neuropsychologization, it's a form of racism.

BB: Absolutely.

RC: Now non-Indigenous Canadians really don't recognize the racism against Native people. They'll tell you, "They're really *that way*." And this way of thinking is buttressed by the psychological sciences, the psychiatric sciences, the educational sciences, if you can call them that.

BB: To touch on the "clinical" for a moment, right now, we are at a particularly frightening juncture when it comes to psychiatry and Native people. I know that in Ontario and I imagine in other provinces too, the mental health industry is saying, "there is rampant mental illness among Indigenous people. We need to provide more psychiatric services." And what really scares me is that to varying degrees, they are joining with Indigenous scholars to do this.

RC: Correct, but I would dispute that the scholars in question are *true* Indigenous scholars. They are a lot of people running around calling themselves Native scholars and it's a name I'd give to almost none of them. What you have in fact is a whole bunch of folk encouraged to sell out their own people, and they don't even know who their damned people are. They have no real connection to an Indigenous form of life.

BB: If I understand you correctly, you are saying, if you are not living the life, if you are not following the ways, then by any meaningful standards, you are not Indigenous.

RC: That's it. And I don't see authentic traditions any more.

BB: Let me tell you where I can get tied in knots. I've had Indigenous colleagues object to the fact that I am critiquing psychiatry, stating that Indigenous people need things like psychiatric drugs, when besides that the drugs overwhelmingly damage, history shows that Indigenous people are among the primary victims of psychiatry.

RC: Exactly. And such scholars have been coopted. And you see it in documents as far back as the Royal Commission Report [see http://www.aadnc-aandc.gc.ca/eng/1100100014597/1100100 014637]. The Royal Commission Report was written largely by social workers. And what did the social workers say? What we need is ten thousand social workers on Indian reserves. Now who would have made that recommendation? I certainly wouldn't.

BB: Only "mental health professionals" or others substantially taken in by the hegemony.

RC: Or by the money made available to them.

BB: And whatever the intention may be, turning to the oppressor as the solution can only lead to disaster.

RC: You have to do the hard work if you are to arrive at answers, and we are not doing that. Actually trying to come to terms with why pathology exists, that's way harder than pretending that there is a little guy inside your head that is responsible for the problems that you face and that what we need to do is to drug him or remove him or coopt him.

BB: To switch the focus just a little, I am very interested in the excellent use you make of the Holocaust to show what happens to Indigenous people. Take a comparison that you often make in response to the call for more self-esteem programs to be delivered to Indigenous people to counter the high Indigenous suicide rate. You say, yes, Indigenous people have a high suicide rates. However, in Nazi Germany, Jews had three times the suicide rate of other German citizens. Does anyone think that the problem in Nazi Germany was low self-esteem and a need for self-esteem counselling?

RC: Yes. The point is: Why would we consider it pathology with Native people when we don't with Jews?

BB: Absolutely. And you often draw on the Holocaust to good effect. It's a brilliant strategy and as a Jew, I cannot but applaud it.

RC: You know, from early years, I read widely about the Holocaust.

BB:	And what really impresses me, you actually read Jean Amery [a survivor generally seen as cynical]. You are the only non-Jew I know who has read Amery.
RC:	(laughter).
BB:	Everyone else prefers to read less angry survivors like Elie Wiesel.
RC:	Something not well known about me that may partially explain this, I'm one eighth Jewish. I'm five eighths Iroquois, two eighths Scottish, and one eighth Jewish. And when I was growing up, my parents made sure that I knew everyone's oppressions. Now from Marx I learnt about the Highland clearances and the destruction of the traditional tribal forms of life of the Scottish people which existed before industrialization. I come by it honestly.
BB:	And it has culminated in a highly sophisticated analysis.
RC:	Well, try to find someone who will say something nice about me in Indian country. Everyone hates me.
BB:	My hunch is that this comes from the fact that you eschew comfortable and comforting concepts like reconciliation. You want justice, and you want fundamental change.
RC:	Right now I am writing a paper on Truth and Reconciliation, calling it a fraud.
BB:	I can understand that. I agree that reconciliation is a flawed concept. Even the truth component is fallacious. If the whole operation is set up—and it is—such that you have no power to subpoena government files, how much of "the truth" are you actually going to be able to find?
RC:	Precisely. Anyway, I am not giving up on any of this. Nor am I stopping my activism. And my activism, incidentally, dates back to when I was five.
BB:	What did you do as a child, Roland?
RC:	Along with my parents and other activists, I walked across the border once a year without stopping at Customs, with of course, the possibility existing of getting arrested or whatever. Now it is only later when it dawned on me: Oh, that was political activism on my part. You know, just by remaining alive while they are oppressing you, you are pushing back.
BB:	A way of conceptualizing resistance, incidentally, which strongly divides Holocaust scholars from each other, with some saying that keeping alive may or may not be resistance, depending on how you accomplish it. But to stick with your words here, they remind me

of the title of one of your books: You wrote a book (Chrisjohn and McKay 2017) with the title "Dying to please you". What was going through your mind when you chose this title?

RC: It's meant to be a shot. So that white people will get it. Yes, we are dying and it's because it pleases you to kill us.

BB: And not because we have "low self-esteem" and not because we have a disease?

RC: Precisely. It's because the policy of Canada toward Indigenous people is genocide. The point is if you are being forced to conform to a form of life which is other than what is natural to you, that's coercion. Which in itself leads to self-damaging behavior. There is a whole list of things that happen. We drop out. We drink. We beat our wives. We fail in numerous ways. And yes, of course, self-esteem is an aspect of that. It is not that we naturally have low self-esteem. It is that everything is so orchestrated that we become convinced there is something wrong with us. And that manifests itself in all sorts of ways. You know nothing "breaks" in just one way.

BB: Which is why all these diagnoses and prognoses are so ridiculous.

RC: Yes, it's like what you say in your PTSD articles [see Burstow 2003, 2005], what psychiatry does is leave out context. They are assuming that the world is fine and normal for everybody, whereas what should be assumed is that it is a dangerous and troubling place. And what is worse, in many situations, and certainly in Native country, it is deliberately so. For all intents and purposes, what they are saying is: Let's make life on the reserve as impossible as we can and then say to the Native people, "Okay, make up your mind. You can live in misery on the reserve or you can conform to what we want you to do. It's your choice." You know, in the Holocaust, some people actually bought their ticket to the concentration camp. They purchased a ticket to Auschwitz. Now, the fact that you bought a ticket to go to Auschwitz, does that mean that you agreed with the policy? The choices people are being allowed are on the same level as the choice one might make in response to someone telling you: "I can saw off your arms or I can saw off your leg. Which one?" And they do that to us Indians over and over. And what with the layers of hegemony which cover up what is happening, understandably, people fall for it.

BB: You know, Roland, when I looked at the title of your book on Indigenous suicide, I'm also aware of another dimension that is important in understanding the oppression. As in: What happens

24 B. BURSTOW

to a people like Indigenous communities who are into accommo-
dation, who are into non-interference when they find themselves in
interaction—including forced interaction—with people into
exploitation. If you are dying to please and you are under the auspices of a group set on exploitation, death on some level or other is
likely to result.

RC: Obviously, nothing good can happen. What adds to the problem,
many Indigenous people today have no real grasp of what their
roots are and how we operated. Now it was always the case that we
contended with one another, but the Iroquois weren't trying to
turn everyone into Iroquois and the Cree weren't trying to turn
everyone into Cree. And I think that understanding the political
economics is critical and understanding Marx is helpful. The point
is, whatever we were, we weren't capitalists. And when you look at
how capitalism functions, then you see that whatever we were, it
was under attack. So how to initiate a praxis is the hard part of
resistance. How do you get around this? You know, colonial history is one of insinuation. "Here's a metal pot. Isn't that better
than boiling things in a wooden one?" they tell us. Well, yes, it is,
but you take this, it comes with strings attached. Now left to our
own devices, we both maintained and innovated. That's one of the
lies attached to modern social science. They've lured Native people
into believing that culture is tradition and nothing but that.
Whereas, as Zygmunt Bauman (2014) clearly points out in his
book *Culture as Praxis*, culture is the innovative mechanism also.
It is the balance between the two. But factors like this are left out
of the analysis. And so we can't resist because we've forgotten what
our ancestors knew. And that was how to change things in accor-
dance with circumstances. How do you introduce a television set
and stay Iroquois? Well, you know, if we had the time, we could
have sat down and worked it out. We could have done that easily.
All First Nations could have. Now the problem I've run into over
and over again is that most everyone thinks it's a psychological
process of some sort. It's not. Go back to classical Marx on this
one. It is not the consciousness of agents that determine society. It
is the society which determines consciousness. What goes along
with this, people have to understand colonization as an economic
phenomenon. As soon as you separate workmanship from
ownership, you have altered the form of life. The very essence of

humanity has been denied. You have drastically changed the relationship between human beings and nature. Anyway, you have in Indian country people saying, "We have to get with the program. This is the twenty-first century. And we can be Indians and still invest and be capitalists and work nine-to-five jobs, etc." But they don't see that there is a connection between the way that the political economy in which they are enmeshed is structured and what is happening to us psychologically. They are acting as if the psychology comes first, and they think, let's correct the psychology and then people will get better. And Marx even knew better than that. He said, let's change the political economy and then we'll see what happens.

BB: I get your point. To go to a related point, what do you think of the early schisms between the Marxist movement and the anarchist movement?

RC: I have to come down on the side of the Marxists. The issue is the depth of the analysis. Now to be clear, we don't have to agree with the Marxist solution. Myself, I really don't agree with the developmental sequence Marx insists on. We were perfectly "in order" as we were. And this is something Marx discovered at the end of his life and you find it in the ethnological notebooks [see https://www.marxists.org/archive/marx/works/1881/ethnographical-notebooks/notebooks.pdf], when he realized that the people he was calling barbarian had a better grasp of how to make a society work than we do. That said, I am anarchist in the following way: I think that civilization as we know it is all going to fall apart and if we survive at all, that small communities will emerge because those are a lot more functional. Which brings me back to the problem of methodological individualism. To assume that different levels of analysis are related to one other, my!

BB: And this is how we end up with reductionism.

RC: Yes. And again, conceptual analysis is not an empirical process. Now to be clear, I think Indians believed in methodological individualism as much as any western capitalist did. We believed that your individual behavior was somehow the result of your internal contents, okay? But the thing is that we did not have a political economy which made this obviously untrue. In other words, if you grew corn, it was the corn that *you grew*, that *your people grew*. It is not like Nike where you have no idea where they came from and the kind of misery that you inflict on the world in the process of producing or using it. We lived in a much smaller world in a political economic sense, and in such a world, it makes more sense to say things like: "You did what you did because you were not acting well as a person." Which contrasts with: you did that because the downturn of the dollars created the following situation in the Greek economy, and so on and so forth. Our societies were not complicated in the way that capitalism has managed to complicate them. And so I am looking to the day, if we survive long enough, when our societies are going to be a lot more local and self-directed, and necessarily anarchist. A friend once asked me if there is a political philosophy that summarizes the Iroquois way, what is it? And my answer is that the Confederacy was an anarchy—a bottom-up anarchy. But it was a well-managed one, which is why it was successful. Now Marxism is useful because it analyzes the system that we are currently stuck with—and that's one that we don't understand. And it's that one that we are continually psychologizing and psychiatrizing, and neuro-philosophizing, with everyone talking about it as if it were a brain process of some sort. And again, it is the Wittgensteinians who are leading the philosophical fight against that entire notion. It is philosophically illegitimate.

BB: Understood. Now Roland, you have been waging the fight you are about largely in academia. What other avenues do you see for resistance?

RC: Well, you have to live it—obviously. And I can honestly say that I grow about half my food.

BB: Where exactly are you located?

RC: Find the most empty spot in New Brunswick, stick a pin in it—and that's us—Lower Jemseg. Now it is a dead end—no easy way in or out—but a dead end where no one uses artificial fertilizers, nor has in living memory. So the land is good, unlike on my own reserve, where you cannot even drink the water.

BB: You know, I talked to an Indigenous colleague but a few days ago who tells me that he just visited his reserve; and there is a doctor there who has most everyone on psychiatric drugs. What might be done about that?

RC: Unfortunately, that is happening everywhere. I've seen it too. Now I am big on the Iroquois way of handling problems: That is, if you are doing the wrong thing or you think someone else is, assume that they are not doing it out of malice but because they don't know. So I have always prioritized education as a form of activism—by which I mean *real education*, not the phony stuff that is going around—and *advocacy for real education*. We do believe in methodological individualism and so our strategy is a bottom-up one. Make a more thoughtful child and you will produce a more thoughtful adult eventually—and they will create more thoughtful adults. But it has to be done personally. And people have to understand the connection between their actions and how they world reacts to that. You know, on a related point, everyone wants to talk about Indians as hunters and gatherers. And I teach against that. What I tell my students is that your ancestors were as agricultural as anyone. I even bring their corn into class and say: See, this is the corn that your people grew and they grew this kind because you had a shorter growing season and you needed smaller corn, but you liked the corn that the Iroquois were growing and so you grew a shorter version of it that took a month less. And they didn't know this. They didn't understand that wild rice is just something cultivated differently than western people would cultivate it. So some of our Nations moved around because we knew what was happening where and when it was happening. And how did they know that? Because they had set it up to be that way. Everyone was an agriculturalist and Natives today need to understand that. And the lies that Indigenous people have been told about themselves are getting in the way of people doing more reasonable advocacy and actions. So what I try to do is help students understand their history, understand what colonization actually is; stress the critical importance of de-psychologizing, and encourage them get back to the old authentic tradition—which included resistance. Make no mistake about it, we were a people given to resistance. As thoughtful adults who knew who we were, we would not put up with that stuff that they were spewing at us, which is why they came for the children. The reason is that the children could not intellectually defend themselves. That's why they were the target.

BB: I think you are absolutely right. My sense is there are other reasons too—first because they are the future, and I'm sure we agree on this, and the second is—and correct me if you think I am way off—I think they also came for the children because if you remove a child from an organic society, everyone's role suddenly disappears and the whole society starts to collapse.

RC: Yeh. And what they figured out is that "Indians as Indians" were unstoppable. So we needed to be turned into something else. And the thin edge of the wedge is the imposition of European technologies, where we took up things which were on one level superior but would not endure in the climates in which we lived. So when I teach, I stress that you need to understand the difference between what looks useful and where it may lead to in the long run, also the difference between what you yourself choose and what is forced upon you.

BB: Otherwise, you are just robbed of a way of living that makes sense. And you end up beholden to the very people who are robbing you.

RC: And you are ripped off. You know, Nikes have less of a markup than the pelts in the fur trade were.

BB: A point well taken. Do keep up your resistance, Roland. Keep up your authentic education.

RC: And I should add, besides education, I believe in direct activism. You know, in the 1970s, I was part of the American Indian Movement in Canada. We had a farm. We had a survival school. And we were listening to police calls so we would appear when the London City Police Force were finding a drunken Indian to beat up. Here's how that worked: There was a code that went out. And everyone would come to kick the Indian. We would show up with a camcorder and start asking questions. That's as in-your-face activist as you can get. But where are these people now? We should have been activists all along. And we're not.

BB: How to shift that is a humongous question. Now correct we if I am wrong, but my sense is that you hold very little hope for things changing.

RC: Very little hope at all. But I still do what I can. Now when people ask me for my advice, I say: Become as much a generalist as you can. You see that's the distinction between living under capitalism and living in a society where workmanship is not separate from ownership. When you are a full human being, you are engaged in all the activities to live as a human being. So I say, if you want to survive, find things that facilitate survival. Some of my students have become midwives, for example. Now I don't think that the people with the big guns are going to go gently into the night when everything starts to fall apart. Nonetheless, we need to try. And that means not following the rules of separation of workmanship. And it means being a whole lot better than we have ever been trained to think of ourselves as being. You have to know the philosophy. You have to know the mathematics. You have to know the seed culture. And rather than planning for sustainability, which is an impossible goal, we need to plan for sufficiency. And that's really what Iroquois culture was all about—sufficiency. What do we need to get by? So you grow your own food and so forth. So the questions I tell students that we need to ask are: How do we get clothes? What are the medications that we really need, as opposed to the bogus psychiatric ones? And if you don't think this way, then you are dependent. Capitalism has turned you into its slave, which is why you think it is so difficult to be otherwise. I don't know whether this is anarchist, or Iroquois, or some combination of the two. The idea, anyway, is to put together what capitalism has pulled asunder. And in the process, to find again what the psych disciplines have rendered invisible.

BB: Which brings us to the close of our interview—and much thanks for the wisdom you have bestowed on us today. Roland, is there anything that you would have liked me to ask you that I haven't?

RC: Hmmm…As far as I can see, you've asked pretty much everything.

BB: Thank you again.

References

Baker, G., & Hacker, P. M. S. (1980/2014). *Understanding and meaning: Volume one of an analytical commentary on the Philosophical Investigations* (2nd ed.). New York: Wiley.

Bauman, Z. (2014). *Culture as praxis.* London: Sage.

Burstow, B. (1992). *Radical feminist therapy.* Newbury Park: Sage.

Burstow, B. (2003). Toward a radical understanding of trauma and trauma work. *Violence Against Women, 10*(11), 1293–1317.

Burstow, B. (2005). A critique of posttraumatic stress disorder and the DSM. *Journal of Humanistic Psychology, 45*(4), 429–445.

Chrisjohn, R., & McKay, S. (2017). *Dying to please you.* Penticton: Theytus.

Representative Publications of Roland Chrisjohn

Chrisjohn, R. (1991). Faith misplaced: Lasting effects of abuse in a first nations community. *Canadian Journal of Native Education, 18*(2), 161–197.

Chrisjohn, R., and Associates. (2008/2017). An historic non-apology, completely and utterly not accepted: A response to Harper's statement of June 11, 2008. Web-published pamphlet, published June 12, 2008; reproduced in Chrisjohn, R., & McKay, S. (2017). *Dying to please you: Indigenous suicide in contemporary Canada.* Penticton: Theytus.

Chrisjohn, R., & McKay, S. (2019). *"And Indians, too:" indigenous peoples and the Canadian form of racism*. Vernon: John Charlton Publishing.

Chrisjohn, R., & McKay, S. (2017). *Dying to please you: Indigenous suicide in contemporary Canada*. Penticton: Theytus.

Chrisjohn, R., & Peters, M. (1986). The right-trained Indian: Fact or fiction? *Journal of American Indian Education, 25*(2), 1–7.

Chrisjohn, R., & Wasacase, T. (2009). Half-truths and whole lies: Rhetoric in the 'apology' and the truth and reconciliation commission. In G. Younging, J. Dewar, & M. DeGagné (Eds.), *Response, responsibility, and renewal: Canada's truth and reconciliation journey*. Ottawa: Aboriginal Healing Foundation.

Chrisjohn, R., & Young, S. (1994/1996/2002). *The circle game: Shadows and substance in the Indian residential school experience in Canada*. Penticton: Theytus.

Chrisjohn, R., Towson, S., & Peters, M. (1988). Indian achievement in schools: Adaptation to hostile environments. In J. Berry, S. Irvine, & E. Hunt (Eds.), *Indigenous cognition: Functioning in cultural context* (pp. 257–283). New York: Springer.

Chrisjohn, R., Towson, S., Pace, D., & Peters, M. (1989). The WISC-R in a native application: Internal and external analysis. In J. Berry & R. Annis (Eds.), *Ethnic psychology: Research and practice with immigrants, refugees, native peoples, ethnic groups, and sojourners*. Amsterdam: Swets & Zeitlinger.

Chrisjohn, R., Wasacase, T., Nussey, L., Smith, A., Legault, M., Loiselle, P., & Bourgeois, M. (2002). Genocide and Indian residential schooling: The past is present. In R. Wiggers & A. Griffiths (Eds.), *Canada and international humanitarian law: Peacekeeping and war crimes in the modern era*. Halifax: Centre for Foreign Policy Studies, Dalhousie University.

Roland's Added Comment

I'm compelled to add that, as well as Ludwig Wittgenstein, Karl Marx, Nancy Fraser, and Peter Hacker, an important contributor to my thinking as has been the great scholar and public advocate, Rajeev Bhargava, whose work, *Individualism in social science*, has, for more than 20 years now, been required reading for all my advanced students. The writing of Michael Maraun, a former student that left me coughing in his dust eons ago, I also consider fundamental to getting past the obfuscation of the modern academic pseudo-sciences. And, as mentioned in the chapter, my time spent with Thomas Szasz, first in his writing and then in a brief but intense first-person encounter, was essential to clearing up muddles in my own head. His works remain important to anyone trying to understand the oppressive (and intentional) impediment mainstream psychiatry and psychology constitutes to a clear understanding of Native predicaments today. (You don't have to agree with his politics, though!) Lastly, I must once more express my surprise that Dr. Burstow managed to find me. I can only imagine that I must thank Brenda LeFrançois for more than just her book (edited with Bonnie Burstow and Shaindl Diamond), *Psychiatry disrupted* (2014), which has helped me keep current.

CHAPTER 3

"Our Freedom of Speech Over Our Medical License": Dialogue with "The Conscience of Psychiatry"—Peter Breggin

An "honorable psychiatrist" and a meticulous researcher, Peter Breggin has authored hundreds of publications which scientifically demonstrate the fraudulent nature of psychiatry's claims. There is a one-to-one correlation, demonstrates Peter, between the purported therapeutic effects of a psychiatric treatment and the degree to which it damages the brain. Related activities of Peter's include hosting a radio show, managing a huge resource center website (www.breggin.com), and serving as an expert witness in courts of law. If you have time to read but one scientific book in this area, do consider picking up Peter's groundbreaking work Toxic Psychiatry.

Peter and I have been close allies since the early 1980s. Correspondingly, despite very real political differences, we are joined together in our goals with respect to psychiatry and in a bond of friendship, mutual support, and respect.

BB: Nice to be talking to you, Peter. I am aware as I ponder your career—and you've been an absolute leader in the fundamental critique of psychiatry, something not even your worst critics could deny—that you have become progressively more radical over the years. I remember back in the early 1980s when us activists were calling for the abolition of electroshock, while you were supporting us, you were somewhat taken back that we were asking that it be

© The Author(s) 2019
B. Burstow, *The Revolt Against Psychiatry,*
https://doi.org/10.1007/978-3-030-23331-0_3

33

34   B. BURSTOW

       abolished, though eventually, you yourself moved to the position of ECT abolition. Would you like to say something about that transition?

PB: It's not exactly more radical. What it was is that I was more libertarian in the beginning. I had in a good way been under the influence of Thomas Szasz, who was fundamentally libertarian. And for a little while in the early 1970s, I was also working in the libertarian political movement. And I was very much upfronting freedom as the first value. And that is the basic principle of libertarianism—voluntary relationships. And I came to see that to some degree, that was utopian. It did not take into account the extraordinary abusive influences that psychiatrists have on their patients when their patients so-called voluntarily agree to electroshock. What I could see is that hardly any patient ever *genuinely* agreed to electroshock—I never saw a case where they had a serious discussion with the doctor about the brain-damaging effects.

BB: Nor are there any cases where they are given honest information.

PB: Precisely. So that simply became more apparent to me. Which is similar to what had happened to me earlier around lobotomy. The point is that unless someone wanted to kill or badly injure themselves, they would not knowingly submit to electroshock or lobotomy. You know, I was actually attacked by Thomas Szasz when I called for the abolition of lobotomy.

BB: There's one of Szasz's major failings—he thought in terms of an imaginary free market in which lobotomies and other "treatments" could be freely chosen and so be okay.

PB: That's it. Yes, for sure, it's an imaginary free market when involuntary treatment hangs over your head and you're too depressed to defend yourself. Anyway, he wrote in a footnote that people who want to abolish lobotomy are worse than the lobotomists.

       Thomas, he just didn't connect very well, Bonnie.

BB: Despite the enormity of his contribution—and it is hard to overestimate it—there is something incredibly deficient about his analysis. And this is an example.

PB: There is. *Real people* are missing from his thinking.

BB: The people, the humanity, and some of the politics. He understood certain aspects of the politics involved brilliantly, for instance, that the diseases are manufactured for the purposes of the psychiatric industry—but he did not understand that insofar they are

3 "OUR FREEDOM OF SPEECH OVER OUR MEDICAL LICENSE"... 35

manufactured by a profession which lies yet is granted huge credibility, you cannot ever have free and informed consent.

PB: I agree with you. You know, I was very active in libertarian conferences for a time, was actually on the board of directors of the Libertarian Party. But then I realized that the fundamental concept of a voluntary exchange was utopian. And I gave a talk clarifying that we cannot just say that we favor voluntary exchange because in every exchange someone has the upper hand. People do not enter what is called voluntary exchanges with equal power. So the concept is problematic. This notwithstanding, much to the chagrin of most people in the antipsychiatry movement, I remain a pretty conservative libertarian, basically small government. I am against "big everything".

BB: I can surely relate to that as an anarchist.

PG: You know, I was one of the first people to look inside the inner workings of the drug companies—and what I found was appalling. What was clear is that nowhere was there a conscience. All the efforts were to make a profit and to protect the product.

BB: For sure, and to market it. What we are looking at is a huge sales job. And you cannot have consent when someone is doing a "snow job" on you—and even less so when you're desperate.

PB: I would add, of all the drug company memos that I've ever encountered, I almost never saw one when people were expressing concerns about the drugs, about the importance of being more cautious.

BB: Let me ask you a somewhat different question. You call yourself—and with good reason—the conscience of psychiatry. But to problematize the word, is it possible for psychiatry to have a conscience when it's based on fraud?

PB: I don't think that psychiatry can ever have a conscience. The profession cannot look at the truth quite simply because the truth is that psychiatry's very basis is fraudulent, is unscientific, is unfounded. The basis being first that more or less all human suffering that seems to be psychological is biologically and genetically determined. And the second part of it is that it can be treated with biological agents. And that isn't true either.

BB: If I might ask you about Gøtzsche, the Danish doctor Peter Gøtzsche [see https://www.madinamerica.com/author/pgotzsche)], theorizes psychiatry as a criminal enterprise. Do you agree with that depiction?

PB: I am going to let *him* continue with the stronger language. That said, there is no doubt that the drug companies and psychiatry will use almost any means to accomplish their ends, and in that way, they very much resemble a criminal conspiracy. For example, an awful lot of what goes on in psychiatry involves leaders in psychiatry taking money from, receiving favors from the drug companies in a cycle which affects all of prescribing throughout the world. And much of it contains criminal conspiracy elements. And the federal government has found some of these companies not only guilty of fraud but of criminal activity.

BB: Which corruption is common and absolutely horrific, though not even close to the totality of what is wrong with this industry. Okay, Peter, change of topic for what I hoping to zero in on in this book is not so much what's wrong with psychiatry as how to combat it. So let me ask you some questions more directly focused on that issue. How do we proceed? Do you think, for example, that The Convention on the Rights of Persons with Disabilities [see http://www.un.org/disabilities/documents/COP/crpd_csp_2017_3.pdf] and the various recent statements by the U.N. can be of any help to us in reining in psychiatry?

PB: No, because I don't trust the UN at all. The UN is in the pockets of some of the greatest negative influences forces on earth and it has always encouraged drug use around the world. Look at the WHO [World Health Organization] studies that backfired on them [studies on the use of antipsychotic drugs pioneered by UN that did not prove the success of the drugs that they were intended to prove; for a discussion of these, see Whitaker 2010].

BB: But we're talking about completely different instruments of the UN. The World Health Organization, yes, is dedicated to whatever they call help, which alas, means pushing drugs. By contrast, the Convention is dedicated in large part to protecting people from interference, including psychiatric interference. And to bring in yet another instrument, a number of UN rapporteurs on torture have declared involuntary psychiatric treatment a form of torture [for details, see http://www.chrusp.org/home/psychiatric_torture]. We have likewise seen official interpretations of the Convention by UN committees concluding that judges throughout the world should be ordering psychiatric institutions to remove the locks from wards and to inform residents that they are free to leave.

3 "OUR FREEDOM OF SPEECH OVER OUR MEDICAL LICENSE"... 37

That's a very different thing than the World Health Organization and their studies.

PB: To be honest with you, I haven't looked into these instruments of the UN, and that's partly because I fear the UN politically more than I praise it. Personally, I think all of these huge organizations are terrible.

BB: That may well be, but the justice system is likewise a large and problematic complex, and yet we all of us include using the court as part of our strategy.

PB: I don't want the US to be controlled by the UN.

BB: I don't see any possibility of that. But let me ask you something: If the UN found the States guilty of human rights violations against psychiatric survivors, you don't think that just might be helpful as leverage?

PB: I haven't thought much about it, Bonnie. Bottom line, I don't want the UN having any power over the United States.

BB: How about the power of influence? You know, a lot of people are using UN pronouncements now as leverage, including in the survivor movement.

PB: Well, the survivor movement as a group has a different political philosophy from me. You know, I wrote a book called "*Wow, I'm an American!*" [Breggin 2009] in which I discuss how the founding principles of this nation are shining lights to the world. I don't believe that is true about the UN.

BB: The founding principles aside, do you, for instance, not see the US as an imperialist power?

PB: Not the way left-wingers see it. I'll tell you what I do think. Human nature is flawed and the larger and more powerful any institution is, the more corrupt it is. And we are in a very bad situation now where the giant corporations from the oil companies to Google are running things and creating massive problems.

BB: They surely are.

PB: And that is a really serious problem, but it is not a uniquely American problem.

BB: No, though America is more deeply implicated in global capitalism than most other countries.

PB: In some ways, but I see things differently. You know, I start with the freedom of the individual. Now I was very much a leftist in my early years, in high school and so on.

BB: I didn't know that.

PB: What I realized when I was doing therapy was that I was supporting entirely the individual in front of me. And I was encouraging the individual to take full responsibility for every choice and reaction in their lives. It didn't mean you don't look at circumstance—I was always a feminist from very early on. So of course, I would look at the influences as I saw them. I was very aware of racism and economic differences. With my wife Ginger, I wrote *The War Against Children of Color* [see Breggin and Breggin 2002] and crushed a giant eugenic program that was brewing. But my emphasis has always been to live one's life by the most ethical, rational, loving principles you can and to take full responsibility not to harm other human beings and to make the most of your own life. And I gradually began to feel that this did not fit with the leftist philosophy which I had, that left-wing philosophy was much more a victimology. And I should say that when I started to take on the lobotomists and sought help, no leading liberal in Congress or the Senate would support me with the exception of the Black Caucus, though the conservatives did. That's the problem with being a liberal, you never get to know conservatives. So I got to know some conservatives and some libertarians and they supported me and they asked me my philosophy and I told them; and they said: That's not liberal. That's conservative (laughing).

BB: I surely do get that. You also, though, have a huge following on the left, correct?

PB: I do, but I have also been badly attacked by the left. And to be clear, the attacks from the right are not even close to what happens from the left. The right has mainly supported me. And why do they support me? Because I talk about individuals. Because I talk about families, and they understand that what psychiatry does interferes with family values and responsibility.

BB: Got it.

PB: I have been invited onto many conservative radio programs to talk about the drugging of children. I have never been invited onto a liberal show about it.

BB: I am not denying the distinction you are making as for sure the left has been problematic when it comes to psychiatry. But you know, if I look at the various US presidents, whether they be democrat or republican, they've all pushed psychiatry.

PB: That's right, Bonnie. Nonetheless you may be shocked to learn that some of the most important help that I got in my campaign to ban psychosurgery was from an extreme conservative in the Nixon Whitehouse.

BB: Though I am a leftist, what you're saying actually doesn't surprise me because I've always known that overall the right wing has been more concerned than the left with protecting the individual, which is one of the reasons I am a left-wing anarchist rather than a Marxist. And I have always understood that when it comes to stopping psychiatric intrusion, there are important allies on the right.

PB: The groups that I have received the most support from have been feminists, people on the right, and African Americans.

BB: Yes, and I can see how that happens. Now my guess is that given the individualistic emphasis, you get little if any support from the Indigenous community—but correct if I'm mistaken.

PB: I don't have contact with them at all.

BB: Because the individualist emphasis would run counter to Indigenous belief systems, to the need to attend to "all our relations".

PB: Let me just say this. The older I get, the more I've come to understand that relationship is what life is about. But, to be clear, conservatives deeply believe that. They believe in family, extended family, church, community. So conservatives understand when I talk about relationship being the center of life.

BB: There is no question that once you enter the area of psychiatry that politics as many of us normally understand it does not apply.

PB: Agreed. It gets enormously confusing.

BB: That said, I want to go back to something you touched on earlier. My sense—and my guess when I look at the trajectory of your books and articles is that it is your sense too—is that the biggest threat right now comes from the psychiatrization of children and the danger to posterity which this poses.

PB: I agree. And I also think that it is the one issue that the average person can most easily understand.

BB: Yes, absolutely, which also means that it is here where we have the greatest possibility of allies.

PB: I agree with that too. And I believe that what psychiatry does to children constitutes child abuse.

BB: As do I, and we have both written on this. Actually, I have an article coming out next month (Burstow 2017) and I will be very inter-

40 B. BURSTOW

ested to see what you think of it. Now I quote you extensively in it, but I also quote the UN Convention on the Rights of the Child (http://www.ohchr.org/EN/ProfessionalInterest/Pages/CRC. aspx) in order to demonstrate the fit between giving children psychiatric drugs and the UN's notion of child abuse.

PB: Okay, I don't mind people citing such conventions. However, I do think that if the UN has any control over our politics, that would be the most cataclysmic development in our history.

BB: Be that as it may, what I am looking for is not the UN gaining control but us highlighting the pronouncements they are making about human right violations. The point here is that a major international body that rightly or wrongly is looked to for guidance, has actually named the everyday practice of involuntary psychiatry a human rights violation. Which puts into question some of the worst of what psychiatry routinely does in every single country throughout the world.

PB: Well, that could be very interesting. Who knows? Maybe some good will come of it.

BB: Peter, if we could zero in more tightly on strategy, how do you see us proceeding in a way that will stop the psychiatric violation of children?

PB: Each person who cares needs to find their own creative way and their own group because there are many ways one can go. One way I'm going about it is laying bare the science. And I have been inviting people to look at the fact that we give children psych drugs, whereas we don't give them marijuana, we don't give them alcohol—we consider it a crime. And the routine use of psychiatric drugs are definitely more harmful in the long run than a moderate amount of alcohol.

BB: A good, and I think, useful comparison. And for sure we need to say these things and to cite research backing it up. At the same time, while we make such cases in our books and articles and we all have proven our points a thousand times over, we are not winning the battle. And that's why I am concerned about strategy. Laying bare the facts is essential, I agree. At the same time, it has been shown to be not remotely sufficient as a strategy.

PB: Right. Anyway, it's one thing to do. How about I tell you about the things I do and maybe others will find them useful? Another thing I do is everything in my power to communicate to the public.

3 "OUR FREEDOM OF SPEECH OVER OUR MEDICAL LICENSE"... 41

BB: You sure do, yeah.

PB: I have a website [see https://breggin.com/]. I have frequent alerts which I send out. I am blogging on other peoples' sites, largely Bob Whitaker's site, also a conservative site called "Natural News" which is on nutrition. I don't post any longer on *Huffington Post*, which is left and incredibly pro-psychiatry.

BB: Frighteningly pro-psychiatry.

PB: And again, that's left. And the kids that come on keep critiquing me.

BB: Agreed, though to be clear, they are not the left that I identify with. Which brings me to another topic, those of us who make mileage critiquing psychiatry—and I see you as a giant here—we all get attacked mercilessly in the media, especially by the mainstream media. We are falsely accused of being scientologists. We are falsely accused of being unscientific. How do you see us successfully addressing the problem?

PB: You know, I have had somewhat of a breakthrough around the Michelle Carter case [a case of a woman charged in a court of law where Peter was an expert witness for the defense; see https://breggin.com/the-michelle-carter-case-archive/]. Two weeks ago I was interviewed for 90 minutes by 20/20 and I really had a chance to educate them.

BB: Good to hear.

PB: I believe I changed the whole tone of the show. That was very unusual. It's way harder for me and others to get on the media now than it was twenty years ago.

BB: Incomparably harder. In fact, it wasn't hard at all twenty year ago.

PB: And in the US, it's because the drug companies mostly got the right to engage in direct advertising to the public; and that's largely meant that they became the lifeblood of the media. The other part of the problem is the drug companies' lobbying, and the interconnecting of the boards of directors.

BB: Absolutely. To come back to the issue of strategy, how do we combat it?

PB: We have to appeal directly to the people.

BB: So going more populist? Not a bad idea.

PB: And that's pretty much where my efforts go.

BB: Which for sure leads to social media kind of work.

PB: We do so much social media. I speak, I blog, and so forth. We may even start publishing cheap books.

BB: When you say "we", do you mean yourself and Ginger [Peter's wife]?

PB: Yes (laugher). Yes, everything's Peter and Ginger. It's been that way since 1985. I did a lot before Ginger but very unhappily.

BB: Yes, and you guys make an impressive team.

PB: We are looking into self-publishing, bringing out inexpensive books that people can buy. It breaks my heart to see people at conferences looking at the price of my book on psychiatric drug withdrawal and shaking their head because they cannot afford to buy it. That's another direction. And of course, I have a radio show [see http://drpeterbregginshow.podbean.com]. I am a guest on other people's radio shows. And also, I do the legal work. And the most head-on way that I confront the issues is in the courtroom.

BB: It surely is, and you're excellent at it. And that's a very special opportunity that you and other critical psychiatrists can avail themselves of.

PB: So there's all those different ways. Then the organizations of people who have been injured have things they can do. And there's two different kinds of organizations, as I see it. The ones that are tied into a leftist approach. And then there are those that have had a loved one hurt. And these are a very different groups of people. The second, more conservative and family-oriented.

BB: And sometimes not.

PB: And sometimes not.

BB: And actually, these groups greatly overlap. But either way, I agree, this is a critical group. The centrality of survivors is a given, and we should talk more about that. And at the same time, I have long felt that that it is with parents that one of the greatest promises for a turnabout lie. Why? Because parents are credible to the average person. And they have seen their children injured. And they have seen their children killed.

PB: Yeah.

BB: And we all know lots of stories where the child was put on psychiatric drugs, with the diminishment of their life that resulted being so horrible that eventually, the child killed himself because they didn't have a life any more [for an example, see Burstow 2015, Chapter One].

PB:	And one of my favorite activities is helping children come off these drugs. That said, let me tell you something else about what I'm doing as a way of talking about what we *all* can do. I've teamed up with nutritionist Pam Popper. Pam is a naturopath. And like me, she is completely scientifically based. What she believes in is a diet based on evolution and scientifically documented, which is a plant-based diet. And you can't eat much fat. Gets away from additives, etc.
BB:	Here we have something physical which actually does influence one's moods, one's psychological well being. Which is legitimate and a meaningful direction as opposed to approaches based on bogus mental illnesses.
PB:	Exactly. Now together we have produced a credit college course that is on why and how to stop taking psychiatric drugs. And it will grant a certificate. I have created video presentations. And we are going to move toward trying to teach people how to help themselves and each other, and even to help disturbed people, regardless of any previous degree.
BB:	You mean in part that you are helping them to become first-rate counselors?
PB:	Yes. We will call them something that isn't licensed. So the goal here is to deliver inexpensive counsellor-type help outside of the medical and psychiatric system. So that's another way that I am going about the work.
BB:	All good. So you're focusing more on what used to be called "alternatives".
PB:	Yes. Now other groups have also set up their own therapy certificate programs. But we may be the first to say: We want to be really helpful without anyone having to have such things as degrees.
BB:	Not the first. That greatly factored into the humanist therapy movement during the 70s.
PB:	So Ginger and I are both in accord on this. And Pam and I are working at developing full care clinics where the first line of treatment is nutrition and counseling. And we can provide cheap help that will work and that people can afford.
BB:	I appreciate and support the principle here, but what about people who are homeless? They can't afford *anything*. Nor can most of the working class. Nor can most racialized people. An inevitable problem when employing a private business model.

PB: Pam has actually shown that her diet can easily be done on food stamps—that's the beauty of it.

BB: Wonderful. Though the counseling can't be.

PB: Well, probably not. But if you're the kind of counselor we are talking about, you may be making fifteen, twenty bucks an hour. And maybe some organization will sponsor you. That's our goal—to get counseling into the hands of good honest ethical people, who are in touch with their own emotions, which is not a product of education at all.

BB: It sure isn't. And I like the implicit de-professionalization involved. That said, as for the issue of money, you know, feminist therapists for four decades now have reserved spots for people with very little money. And besides that the therapists have had trouble making ends meet, the tiny bit of money being charged is still too much for legions of people, making us inaccessible.

PB: Nonetheless, you could set up a clinic this way that could provide very inexpensive health care. So there's a whole lot of things I am involved in. I'm doing a lot of good stuff.

BB: Yes, you surely are, Peter. And are you still going to be one of the people trying to stop intrusive state laws being passed? Or will you be leaving that to others?

PB: Which laws?

BB: Say, laws like the ones recently passed, like the outpatient commitment laws and the US legislation that requires all children to be subjected to a psychiatric examination?

PB: Yes, those laws are atrocious, and absolutely I will still speak about it. However, it's not where I am going to be putting my greatest energies.

BB: So what you are doing with Pam Popper, you are feeling this is your niche right now. I'll be following that with interest. Anyway, let me go back to something we touched on earlier. It's great that you have received some favorable publicity with respect to the Carter case especially after having been given such a hard time by the press. But in general, what do you think would be good strategies for dealing with the maligning of critics of psychiatry by the press?

PB: I think that the more "wins" we have, the more likely we are going to get some coverage and indeed some decent coverage. Nonetheless I don't have any easy answer. The coverage that I recently got came

3 "OUR FREEDOM OF SPEECH OVER OUR MEDICAL LICENSE"... 45

as a result of the Michelle Carter case, some negative, and some of it's pretty good. The biggest media of all—20/20—was *very good*. I think it's *partly* because I am a psychiatrist.

BB: While I'm aware that you always do an impressive job, and I in no way want to minimize that, I think it's *a lot* because you are a psychiatrist. As a psychiatrist, you automatically receive a certain credibility.

PB: (laughing). It's why I went to medical school. Actually, my father said he would put me through graduate school. And I said that I wasn't sure what to pursue. And he asked, "Who has the strongest trade union, son?" I answered, "the medical profession." Whereupon he said, "I'll pay for it."

BB: Interesting. That said, we surely need psychiatrists who tell the truth in this fight. And indeed, we have all of us benefited enormously rom your credibility.

PB: That's wonderful.

BB: Incidentally, you've talked about politicians who are and aren't allies. Among the people actually involved in critiquing psychiatry, where do we find the strongest allies?

PB: I tend to look to Great Britain for there are far more of them with a good critique of psychiatry there than exist in North America.

BB: Absolutely true, and at the same time, what we have in North America is a more enlightened survivor movement. While there are exceptions to be sure, more survivors who are politically aware and vocal.

PB: No question.

BB: Actually, though there are some absolutely stellar UK organizations and allies like Speak Out Against Psychiatry and MindFreedom Ireland, together with courageous leaders like Cheryl Prax and Mary Maddock—and thank God for them—much of the survivor movement as far as I can make out, is close to bought-and-sold in certain parts of England. And that worries me for I look to the survivors. More generally, my sense is that survivors as a whole are far more key to winning this fight than professionals are. They are the oppressed. They are the "experts". They are the folk with the lived experience.

PB: I agree. And that's inevitable.

BB: So it's critical that survivors be front and center.

PB: Agreed. And just to carry on with one of the themes of your book, I think the necessary change is eventually going to come from a combination of people who have been injured and speak out and people who learned enough not to go near psychiatry in the first place. Okay, what should we focus on as we draw to a close?

BB: Peter, how about choosing your own focus?

PB: Let me just say that I am hoping that in the future that we will look back on what is going on in psychiatry and psychopharmacology and the insurance companies and the federal agencies and everyone else in regard to psychiatric drugs as something positively bizarre on every level. The thing about the psychiatric complex is that it has involved us in something similar to a Church-centered state. At the same time as exercising all this power over others, psychiatry is a materialist religion in that it takes psychological, spiritual, social, economic—any kind of issue—and treats it as a material matter related to brain-dysfunction. And that is a wholly wrong and indeed evil approach to human beings, and it results in incredible horror. You know, when you objectify a human being and make statements like, "Well, you can't talk to schizophrenics, just give them drugs for they have a chemical imbalance"—that's the ultimate objectification.

BB: Absolutely.

PB: And when you objectify people like that, you strip away empathy and caring.

BB: Yes, and you fall out of identification. You are not really seeing them as the same species you are.

PB: Yes, in essence, you make them alien, and human beings can be very hostile and violent to people whom they perceive as alien. Our guilt, shame, and anxiety is almost entirely limited to family relationships—that is how it evolved, how we got our moral sense. What I have concluded is that guilt, shame, and anxiety almost entirely developed as a way of keeping us from slaughtering each other in the family setting. We needed guilt, shame, and anxiety before we could develop ethics and empathy. However, it does not prevent us from substantially harming anyone that we identify as non-family, as alien.

BB: Which is why we all have to see everyone and everything as family. As Indigenous communities put it, we have to respect existence, relating to everything that is, was, or will be "as all our relations".

3 "OUR FREEDOM OF SPEECH OVER OUR MEDICAL LICENSE"... 47

PB: And to zero in how this plays out in psychiatry, psychiatry alienates itself from its own patients. And that's how we get mass lobotomies in the US. That's why we can drug 20% of boys with just one diagnosis—ADHD. That's how we can end up with a large percentage of women on medications. That's how we subject people to involuntary treatment and incarceration. We are alienating ourselves from other people by how we define them. And this accounts for lobotomy and electroshock. And this accounts for the role of psychiatry in Nazi Germany and the mass murder of the "mental patients" [described in the book *The War Against Children of Color*; see Breggin and Breggin 2002, also on the website www.breggin.com]. And the answer really is that we have to love one another. We have to expand as you said, the human family. And we have to reach out to protect the rights of one another.

BB: I'm really glad you walked us though this part of your philosophy, Peter, for it has taken us into critical existential territory. That said, anything else that you like to say that we haven't touched on?

PB: You know, with the Carter case, I was asked: What's the worst mistake that Michelle Carter made? And my answer was "taking psychiatric drugs." The point is, taking psychiatric drugs will probably be the worst decision of your life.

BB: Good answer. And to turn this around, in ending, I can't avoid the temptation to ask you something similar, for we all err: In your truly admirable life, Peter, what is the worst mistake that you yourself have ever made?

PB: That's easy. Not marrying Ginger when I first met her in 1974.

BB: That's romantic, but knowing how the two of you operate, it is also a whole lot more than romantic. How long did it take you, Peter?

PB: Eleven years. I knew I was in love, but I was so frightened by love that I didn't get together with her for eleven years.

BB: You guys have gotten closer and closer, haven't you? And the strong opposition to psychiatry that two of you have created—it really is a Peter-and-Ginger operation.

PB: Absolutely. And you know, she's been there through thick and thin. And she has always had this courage, intelligence and integrity. She largely headed the campaign to safeguard my medical license [When Peter critiqued psychiatry on the Oprah Winfrey Show, a pro-psychiatry lobby group and the State of Maryland attempted to strip him of his medical license; see http://www.nytimes.com/1987/09/22/science/free-expression-or-irresponsibility-psychiatrist-faces-a-hearing-today.html?mcubz=3]

48 B. BURSTOW

And later when the American AMA ethics committee agreed to drop the case against me as long as I didn't talk to the press about what happened in this case, do you know what Ginger said, what position she took?: "Our freedom of speech over our medical license."

BB: Principled and gutsy! Something both of you have always been. Say hello to Ginger for me. And Peter, thank you for sharing so much of yourself in this interview.

REFERENCES

Breggin, P. (2009). *Wow, I'm an American.* New York: Lake Edge Press.
Breggin, P., & Breggin, G. (2002). *The war against children of color.* Monroe: Common Courage Press.
Burstow, B. (2015). *Psychiatry and the business of madness.* New York: Palgrave.
Burstow, B. (2017). The psychiatric drugging of children and youth as a form of child abuse—Not a radical proposition. *Journal of Ethical Human Psychology and Psychiatry, 19*(1), 65–76.
Whitaker, R. (2010). *Anatomy of an epidemic.* New York: Broadway Paperbacks.

REPRESENTATIVE PUBLICATIONS OF PETER BREGGIN

Breggin, P. (1991). *Toxic psychiatry: How therapy, empathy, and love must replace the drugs, electroshock, and biomedical theories of the "New Psychiatry".* New York: St. Martin's Press.
Breggin, P. (2001a). *Talking back to Ritalin* (rev.). Cambridge, MA: Perseus Books.
Breggin, P. (2001b). *The antidepressant fact book.* Cambridge, MA: Perseus Books.
Breggin, P. (2006). *The heart of being helpful: Empathy and the creation of a healing presence* (rev.) New York: Springer.
Breggin, P. (2008a). *Brain-disabling treatments in psychiatry: Drugs, electroshock, and the psychopharmaceutical complex* (2nd ed.). New York: Springer.
Breggin, P. (2008b). *Medication madness: The role of drugs in cases of violence, suicide, and crime.* New York: St. Martin's Press.
Breggin, P. (2013). *Psychiatric drug withdrawal: A guide for prescribers, therapists, patients and their families.* New York: Springer.
Breggin, P. (2014). *Guilt, shame and anxiety: Understanding and overcoming negative emotions.* Amherst: Prometheus Books.
(For Dr. Breggin's website, see www.breggin.com)

Peter's Added Comment

I decided on my own to use my comment to express my appreciation of Bonnie Burstow. Due to the profound perspective that Bonnie has on all issues pertaining to the field of "mental health" and psychiatry, this was among the most interesting interviews I have been involved in. In addition to her sheer brilliance in analyzing social issues, Bonnie has done some of the most courageous and innovative work in psychiatric reform. Consider her university classes, scientific articles, detailed scientific books, and fictional and dramatic works. Then there is her amazing scholarship fund at the University of Toronto for studies in antipsychiatry—something I supported while never imagining it could actually be done (for more on the scholarship, see Chap. 15). Thanks for the interview, Bonnie; we are grateful for your presence on Earth.

CHAPTER 4

Dialogue with Journalist Extraordinaire: Robert Whitaker

Robert Whitaker is a leading figure in the world of critical psychiatry. An award-winning American journalist, he has received, for instance, the Polk Award for Medical Writing. And he is the guiding force behind the popular blog site Mad in America. *His books include* Mad in America, Anatomy of an Epidemic, *and* Psychiatry Under the Influence.

While one of us is antipsychiatry and one critical psychiatry, Bob and I have profound respect for each other. Correspondingly, I have been writing for his blog Mad in America *for years.*

BB: Bob, including you centrally in this book was absolutely "mandatory". Not only have you written several ground-breaking books and been an award-wining reporter in the area, in more recent years, you have created a very important and popular platform where people from a number of different communities coalesce and engage in much needed debates—of course, I mean the *Mad in America* blog site [https://www.madinamerica.com/]. Let's start here, for that is probably the work for which you're currently best known. So: How did that site come about?

RW: Initially in a serendipitous way: I wrote my second critical psychiatry book, and I started receiving email saying: "I agree with you. So what are we going to do about it?" Now I 'd had this *Mad in America* personal site from the time that I published my book

© The Author(s) 2019
B. Burstow, *The Revolt Against Psychiatry*,
https://doi.org/10.1007/978-3-030-23331-0_4

51

Mad in America (Whitaker 2002)—and I put all my source documents onto that site. Why? Because if you are writing a counternarrative, the question arises: What are your sources? And for me, personally, the most amazing thing was that this counter-narrative can be found right in conventional psychiatry's *own* source documents. So I was reaching out to the larger society with these documents. That was the first thing. The second is: the doctor Mark Foster and survivor Laura Delano approached me asking: Could we blog? So all of a sudden there were two voices—beyond just me. And the minute that happens, you start thinking: There's power in a collection of different voices. Then I started hearing from psychiatrists, family members, psychologists who wanted to get together to review the evidence. That led to the creation of the Foundation for Excellence in Mental Health Care. And even as this was happening, it became evident that there was an abundance of voices out there eager to write. Now we are in January 2012— and Kermit Cole and Louise Putnam said, "Let's do this." Basically, the idea was to have a journalistic type magazine or publication— you remember the old one, it had three columns like a newspaper—that contained critical information about psychiatry, then a group of bloggers with many different experiences, whether they be psychologists, people with lived experience, family members, or psychiatrists, etc., all from their own unique critical perspective. That was the first thing. The second part was unearthing hidden information: we wanted to highlight all the research news that never gets aired because it contradicts the official line.

BB: Hence your standard news and research column in *Mad in America.*

RB: Exactly.

BB: Let me interject here for a moment. In the process, one of the things that you also succeeded in doing, whether intentionally or serendipitously, is creating a space for community and indeed, a whole bunch of communities. It is not just the bloggers. There are people who never blog for you but who nonetheless always respond to blogs. It is as if you have created a home for them.

RB: Yeah, that was one of our goals too. You know, the original tagline for the site was "Science, History, and Community". Why? Because one of the things that has allowed the conventional story to go forward with such success is they have been really good at isolating critics and delegitimizing them. So we formed a platform for people where they could be in community and not feel isolated. And our ultimate mission was to present that community to society at large.

BB: And from my perspective, you've had great success with all of those goals. That said, let's enter into other areas of your work—and we'll come back to the site later. Now, you didn't begin as someone creating a critical psychiatry site. You began as an investigative journalist and you covered the medical beat for *The Albany Times Union*. You are also someone who has received numerous awards—richly deserved, I might add. I'll tell you what I see as unique in how you went about writing what you wrote—and then how about you commenting on my "take"? Initially when you were a reporter covering medicine, you reported medical stories in a similar way that your journalist colleagues did. And how is that? They lose the sense that they otherwise might have that they are supposed to be doing investigative reporting. Anyway, like everyone else, you slipped into this frame. And then somehow, you turned this around. You realized, Oh my God, I cannot treat medicine differently than other areas which I cover. It behoves me as a journalist to subject it to the same political scrutiny. Could you comment on this? Because I see this as an incredibly important turnabout in your trajectory as a reporter.

RB: You're absolutely right. There's a couple of parts to how this came about. One: I didn't come into journalism as a medical reporter or someone expected to cover sciences. I came into this "backdoor". I spent ten years trying to write fiction, okay? I drove a cab—and I worked in prisons, etc. Those experiences made me highly sceptical about many things. And working in Attica prison made me particularly wary of conventional narratives. The point is, there is a conventional narrative about people in prison—and once you work in prison, it completely falls apart. Anyway, I go to the *Albany Time Union* and get assigned to the Science beat—and you're absolutely right. You go into the science beat and the message becomes: You have a new job, which is to interpret science for the lay public.

BB: Which essentially means accepting the line that you're being fed, right?

54   B. BURSTOW

RW: Absolutely. And the operant belief is that science is this higher ethical pursuit—especially, medicine. The doctor in the white coat has been a cherished image for a long time in society. So the thinking is: Politicians are going to lie to you. And businessmen are going to lie to you.

BB: But you can trust the high priests of medicine. At which point, quite simply, you are no longer operating like a journalist.

RW: Yes, yes. That's what happens. And here's the other thing, Bonnie: These people are seen as pursuing a noble calling. Also as existing in a world that you cannot understand—a world of data, of research. It's too complicated, really, for you.

BB: So as best you can, you just try to simplify the message they are delivering to you and then pass that on?

RW: Precisely.

BB: Let me ask you something—because for sure that squares with what I see with reporters on the medical beat, how did you arrive at the point where you said: What's happening to me? I am not any longer acting like an investigative journalist.

RW: I was covering a story on Albany Medical Center's introduction of laparoscopic gallbladder surgery. So I asked the fellow that I'm interviewing, "So how is it going? Are you having any adverse events? Any surprises?" And the guy knocks on wood and says, "Not here." And I said, "What do you mean 'not here'?" And he answers, "Well, *we* haven't lost anybody."

BB: And that's your tipoff that something's being covered up?

RW: Yeah. Suddenly I saw medicine in a new light. Here's what I discovered: In order to compete with each other, all these hospitals wanted to tout that they had this latest surgery—so what I saw was a marketing angle. Then through a Freedom on Information request, I looked into reports of deaths in gallbladder surgery, which normally are quite rare, and I noticed this unmistakable spike. Okay. Why? Why are people dying? Well, then you dig into the training and you find that the people conducting the initial laparoscopic surgeries were going to seminars run by the makers of the equipment, where they did an operation on a pig and then they went back and did it on human beings. In other words, the training was abysmal. And finally, I looked at how the stock prices of the makers of laparoscopic surgery equipment were soaring—and wow!

BB: You started to notice that you were dealing with a business whose decisions were motivated by self-interest—the type of realization that would stand you in good stead later when you found yourself delving into psychiatry.

RW: That's right.

BB: And you also started to notice the huge contradiction between the espoused line and facticity. And my sense is that this is how you ended up writing your books, okay? So to get back to my earlier point about the uniqueness of your books, when I contrast your books on psychiatry with books by other critics, here's what I see: Most books critiquing psychiatry proceed on the basis of what the author knows *has to be* covered. Your books, by contrast, read differently for you enter in differently. Instead of asking what has to be covered, you start off with the contradictions.

RW: Yes.

BB: E.g., they say these drugs are effective. And yet World Health Organization studies show that in countries that don't have these drugs people recover from "schizophrenia" more quickly. How could that be? You ask these types of questions again and again, and your books seem to stem from those questions, those anomalies. The point is, if I may so depict your process, you go about the job of writing books in the area of psychiatry precisely like an investigative reporter.

RW: Yeah. In other words—let's try to figure this out. Let's go through the evidence.

BB: Okay and I think that's the real strengths of your books, especially *Mad in America* and *Anatomy of an Epidemic*. You begin with a contradiction, then walk people through data which shows how this contradiction got created.

RW: You're absolutely right.

BW: If I might touch on something different, one place where there is a profound disagreement within the *Mad in America* community is between the *critical psychiatry* people and the *antipsychiatry* people—something of course important to me as a committed antipsychiatry theorist. This difference between members of the community is quite pronounced. Now both parts of the community figure in the *Mad in America* network. Nonetheless, *Mad in America*'s mission statement is unqualifiedly *critical psychiatry*—that is, it's in the reform camp as opposed to the abolition camp.

RW: Yup.
BB: Let me ask you something. You yourself have positioned yourself in the reform camp. Where exactly do you disagree with antipsychiatry? With what specific propositions or tenets?
RW: You are asking me what my personal thinking is?
BB: Exactly.
RW: Tell me if you disagree with this: As I see it, the difference between critical psychiatry and antipsychiatry is that critical psychiatry has a sense that psychiatry can be reformed, that it's mistaken but not malevolent. And the antipsychiatry position is that the whole thing is a disaster, malevolent, and needs to be abolished, right?
BB: The abolition part, yes, that is the difference. However, I would not call the attribution of malevolence an antipsychiatry position per se. One group is saying that psychiatry can be reformed whereas the other is judging it irredeemable.
RW: Okay, that's a good framework. So one reason that I am not antipsychiatry is because, the very use of the word "antipsychiatry" means that you have an ideology, okay?
BB: Yes, but Rob, *everyone* has an ideology.
RW: Fair enough, but the point is, I don't give a shit about psychiatry.
BB: I get that. And indeed, all of us are only in the struggle because we care about what happens to people. People—not an industry, psychiatric or otherwise. Where psychiatry comes in is that the damage done is done precisely by institutional psychiatry.
RW: Yeah. So I see this . . . Actually, I am sort of "on the fence" here.
BB: That's my sense. That you created a forum that is not "on the fence", that largely comes down on the side of reform—but that you yourself are on the fence.
RW: Yeah, yeah, that's exactly right (laughter). And here's the thing: I feel like from a practical point of view, psychiatry is going to continue, right?
BB: So is your position—there's nothing we can do about it—and so let's not alienate them too much?
RW: Well . . .
BB: Or let's see if we can't move them a bit?
RW: Right. But on the other hand, personally, it seems hopeless. They are not reformable, okay?
BB: (laughter) Okay, there's the contradiction.

4 DIALOGUE WITH JOURNALIST EXTRAORDINAIRE: ROBERT WHITAKER   57

RW: They're utterly close-minded, and really, psychiatry needs to start completely over.

BB: Question: Why do you want to have psychiatry at all? Why put problems in living that are overwhelmingly not medical into the hands of a medical discipline like psychiatry?

RW: Yeah, yeah, but that's not what I believe.

BB: You believe it is medical?

RW: No, I believe that *sometimes* it is medical.

BB: So, Robert, *when* is it medical?

RW: Oh lots of things can lead to psychosis.

BB: I understand and of course, agree, but the point is that these so-called medical diseases that are the province of psychiatry are not diseases and not medical.

RW: Listen, let's take as an example schizophrenia, right? Everyone will agree that there is no discrete thing called "schizophrenia". It's just a catch-all term.

BB: Yes. And that's not how medicine is supposed to operate.

RW: Yeah, yeah, the psychiatric diagnostic system is a disaster, right?

BB: Okay, but the question is: What is gained by preserving the concept and putting doctors called psychiatrists in charge of it?

RW: Oh, I am not necessarily saying that the doctors should be in charge.

BB: What position should they have?

RW: That they should have a voice in it.

BB: And that is because . . .?

RW: Because certain medical conditions can lead to psychosis.

BB: Sure, but we don't need psychiatrists for that. We simply need doctors. Why doctors known as psychiatrists? Obviously, anything that people experience can have medical complications. So having doctors on the sidelines is not a bad idea. That's very different from having a branch of medicine called "psychiatry" that is predicated on the proposition that these problems in living are inherently medical.

RW: Okay, so Bonnie, let's just separate this out. Right now psychiatry, which is a medical "specialty", has dominion over this part of our social lives, right? And in *Psychiatry Under the Influence* [Whitaker and Cosgrove 2015] we say it shouldn't be that way. What is called "mental illness" is a social construct. So you need philosophers. You need sociologists. Certainly, we need people with lived experience. You also need doctors.

BB:	Sure, doctors and ones from many medical areas—but not the bogus area called psychiatry.
RW:	Well, doctors who specialize in the gut, for example. I believe that nutrition *is* important. Exercise is important. Physical health is important. That sort of thing.
BB:	Absolutely.
RW:	So yes doctors who are good at the whole bodily health dimension need to be involved in a social response. And they can identify certain things. We know that for example as Parkinson's Disease develops, it destroys the basal ganglia—and actually that is commonly associated with psychotic features. Okay?
BB:	Excellent. And we want to be able to rule those out.
RW:	Yeah. And so, Bonnie, if we talk about these manifestations of mental difficulties—psychosis, mania, depression—clearly, there are many different pathways to such things. And it is also a reflection of how society operates, whether it is socially just, poverty-ridden, etc. And so we need a social group to think about this.
BB:	Absolutely.
RW:	So what I am saying is that I don't think that doctors should have dominion over this area of our lives. They should be a contributing voice to identify specific illnesses that are real, but also doctors should be able to have some voice in: How do we maintain healthy lives?
BB:	Absolutely, and I have no problem with that. And significantly that does not leave us with academic psychiatry, or indeed, any psychiatry involved. The point is, in the model that you are articulating, psychiatry as we know it is irrelevant. Note, it is a model that necessarily requires *doctors*—not a model that requires *psychiatrists*.
RW:	So there is no need for psychiatric dominion.
BB:	That's a "given". But what you are articulating goes beyond the question of dominion. There is no need for psychiatry at all. There is a need for doctors. And to boot, doctors would only be one of many groups that coalesce to deal with problems in living and of course, they have a role, for there might be medical issues involved.
RW:	Exactly.
BB:	But the point is that for me, if they are not psychiatrists—and nothing that you have said indicates why they should be—that adds up to psychiatry abolition. Of course, there is a role for neurologists. Nutritionists.

RW: Gastroenterologists.

BB: Absolutely, but we would no longer have psychiatry if we went in that direction. Which would be a very interesting shift and in its own way is a version of psychiatry abolition. That said—and I understand that you might disagree—to hone in on a smaller question, you are one of the people skilled at distinguishing good research from bad. And we know that when it comes to psychiatric drugs, research offers little reason for anyone to take them. Research suggests that if they have any effectiveness at all, it is short-lived, and usually even in the short term, it does not outperform active placebo.

RW: Right.

BB: So for example, we find no greater effectiveness for depression with antidepressants than we find with antihistamines. So should doctors be prescribing such drugs? They could prescribe antihistamines with way less damage done.

RW: Should they be prescribing?

BB: Should they be prescribing psychiatric drugs that have been proven to have no greater effectiveness than active placebo while being considerably more damaging?

RW: This is a larger question about how society thinks about medication. So one of the things that you see in the short-term trials is, if you did a scatterplot of responses, even in the short run, there's little evidence of greater symptom reduction in the drug-treated group than the placebo. And the outcomes worsen in the aggregate with all these medications.

BB: And long-term is critical for that is where the short-term leads. Look at the Rappaport study. The people labelled schizophrenic who fared best are the ones who never went on the drugs in the first place [for details and an analysis of the Rappaport study, see https://www.madinamerica.com/2017/05/psychiatry-defends-its-antipsychotics-case-study-of-institutional-corruption/].

RW: Yes. And the drugs are a trap, okay? Because they change your brain and once you are on them, you can't get off. Let me say, though, you are asking me for an opinion on something that I don't want to render an opinion on.

BB: Fair enough, Bob.

60   B. BURSTOW

RW: Let me explain why: I am someone who is supposed to bring the information forth—and then there can be a larger discussion of whether or not we should be prescribing these drugs.

BB: So you don't want to express an opinion on this yourself—I get that.

RW: No, I don't. What I want is the discussion to be informed by as much information as possible, which includes what you just said.

BB: And you have been one of the key people ensuring that this information is available. And let me say, I think that you are making great strides in what you have set out to do. Question: Would you be okay—and it's fine if you're not—expressing a *personal opinion* with the built-in rider that isn't a position that you're actually advocating?

RW: Sure, personal opinion—as long as it is so labelled.

BB: Absolutely.

RW: Do I think that as a society that we should stop prescribing currently approved psychiatric drugs? Yes, in the sense that as a whole, the way they are being prescribed today, they are likely to do more harm than good. And by the way, this is the same conclusion that Peter Gøtzsche reached [a radical Danish doctor who critiques psychiatry and writes for *Mad in America*] and he has a position in society where he is supposed to offer such opinions. And the only reason that I don't draw that conclusion is that it is not my position in society to do so.

BB: Got it.

RW: But if you're asking my opinion? Absolutely, that's what the data shows. And let's remember: Society got along for thousands of years without these drugs. They used herbs, and they may have used drugs as sedatives and so forth, but they did not have psychiatric drugs that were said to be antidotes for specific diseases. It's that mistaken conception that leads to their misuse and makes them so problematic for society. And so when people say we couldn't do it—Please! The first psychiatric drugs came out in 1955—and society did okay before that. So clearly, we could get along just fine without them. And indeed, if we stopped prescribing such drugs, that would force us to think about other ways to help people. It might even force us to think about what is wrong with society that we have so many folk struggling. It might make us think about how to raise our children so that we don't diagnose

20% of them. So what is my opinion? That we as a society would be *much better off* if we just started over and stopped prescribing these drugs, at least in the way as they are prescribed right now as treatments for a "disease".

BB: Very clear. Okay, I am going to ask you another question in the same general realm. One thing that always worries me about reform, whether we are talking about moral treatment or psycho-analysis, is that historically, the push for reform arises because of a crisis in psychiatry; then psychiatrists themselves climb aboard the reform bandwagon and for a while—sometimes a long while—the reform taking place moderates what is happening to people in distress; it puts a bit of a break on biological psychiatry for biological psychiatry is no longer the norm. And then without fail, a reversal sets in—and biological psychiatry, in short, returns with a vengeance. And so my sense is that reform that is not fundamental simply squanders the momentum for real change. For we end up right back on the same trajectory. Which is one of the reasons that I am very sceptical about reform as opposed to abolition movements. Could you comment on how you see this?

RW: Oh gosh!

BB: I know that these are really hard questions.

RW: No, no, they're really *good* questions. I just want to go back to one thing—I do believe that there are individuals that find these drugs helpful.

BB: Absolutely. And I don't know that a single person in the antipsychiatry movement has called for these drugs being made illegal any more than any of us want to restrict people's access to *any* of drugs that folk use in coping—whether they be psychiatric drugs, or heroine, crack, etc.

RW: Right. And so we all acknowledge that some people have that experience and no one's trying to deny that experience.

BB: Quite right.

RW: To step back, there is something more fundamental than the drugs, and that's that the DSM has been revealed as a failure in every way.

BB: Ah, but to people "in the know"—not to the general public, not to the government.

RW: Yes, but psychiatrists themselves know it has failed; and this goes to your point. And now they are saying maybe they were wrong about their serotonin theory of depression.

BB:	And here is where simplistic reform creeps in. Let's say they make some concessions and let's say reformers are able to put the reins on biological psychiatry. This looks like a promising development. But if we heed the lessons of history, we know that these concessions are short-lived. Reforms are made and then biological psychiatry returns with a vengeance some thirty-forty years later. Why let this happen when we have them on the ropes now? So that's my concern here.
RW:	Yeah, you know where this battle is being fought now? In the adoption of Open Dialogue [mode of psychiatry that is more social]. Because you know how it's being adopted? As a therapy. So in that way, they are "having their cake and eating it too"—it is just a new therapy.
BB:	You are speaking of cooptation?
RW:	Yeah. And it *is* being coopted.
BB:	Which is why I don't think non-abolitionist reform is the more "practical" direction, if I may use that term—though I can certainly see why others think so.
RB:	Look, Bonnie. Put this down to my opinion only, okay?
BB:	Absolutely.
RW:	Do I think psychiatry is reformable? No, not in a big picture way. And that is because: a) so much power is vested in academic psychiatry and in drugs, and in the whole NIMH [National Institute of Mental Health] story and societal authority—and b) because a large part of psychiatry's function in society is about social control. So, we need to have a "revolution". We need to start over. Really, you have to understand the history of psychiatry—that you had these asylums, and then all of a sudden doctors took control of the asylums in 1844; and those doctors really expanded their authority and extended their domain into the community, right?
BB:	While making everything look more and more medical.
RW:	Yes.
BB:	And competitively, driving out all competitors—women especially.
RW:	Yes. And that history is the story of a failed medical specialty. Okay?
BB:	Yes, failed in terms of any validity and any goodness to the world—not in terms of serving itself, in which it greatly succeeded.
RW:	And what they have managed to do time and time again even as they lose credibility and legitimacy, is continue to expand their

empire. Now they are our society's philosophers. They control what we think about ourselves.

BB: And how we think about anyone who disagrees with us?

RW: Exactly, and how we even think about children.

BB: And that's the cruellest cut of all. Children no longer have a chance to have a childhood because psychiatry has in essence redefined regular childhood as a disease.

RW: That's right. And this labeling of children is horrid. The whole point of being alive is coming to grips with one's own mind. So given that, Bonnie, back to your question about reform movements, and you can see this in the two books I wrote. The first book—*Mad in America* [Whitaker 2002]—is really a story about the history of a failed medical speciality. And *Anatomy of an Epidemic* [Whitaker 2010] is the story of the failed DSM-III. Also a failed psychopharmacological adventure. And evident in both histories is that psychiatry as a medical specialty is deluded. It does not know its own history. And it is so deep into its own propaganda it can't see itself. So, can an institution like that reform itself? No, you have to remake everything. And not just the institution. You have to remake the whole societal response to how we care for ourselves and each other. Which reminds me: Can I give you a quick vignette?

BB: Please.

RB: When vacationing in Martinique, at 8:00 a.m. I saw the school bus pull up on this beautiful beach, and the kids from the school jump in this water and swim for about an hour. And they are screaming with delight. And my first thought was: If you start the day this way, I'll bet you don't have ADHD. So what does this vignette show? How society itself creates problems that psychiatrists then "treat".

BB: It surely does. That said, let's return to where we started this conversation—with the issue of journalism. If we look at some of the players involved in the supremacy of psychiatry, we know that a huge part of the problem is coming from the pharmaceutical companies, similarly, the ECT industry. We know that government is part of the problem. We likewise know that a particularly large part is academic psychiatry, which has all this credibility which it uses to sell stories that are not true. Okay. At this point in time, another huge problem is the media itself. The media circulate these stories.

The media dismisses the critics of psychiatry in sensationalistic ways, and far from setting off on their own journeys of discovery, they more or less regurgitate the medical line—with almost the best that we can ever get from them being a story about "over-medicating". Do you have anything to say to your colleagues in the media on how they are handling psychiatry and what they might do differently?

RW: Well, in many ways, I got excommunicated. I can't write about this in the mainstream media because I am seen as biased.

BB: And "biased" means not parroting the standard line?

RW: Right. You know, the *Boston Globe* ran a review of *Anatomy* that likened me to an AIDs denier. And this in some ways is the big problem, for the media serve as a liaison between . . .

BB: Institutional psychiatry and the general public?

RW: Yes. It becomes the vehicle for how the "mental illness" story is told. And the American Psychiatric Association and the pharmaceutical industry join together to use the Scientology slur to make journalists afraid. This was done in the early 90s really effectively. What happens is that journalists see they are going to get attacked if they go down the line of advancing a counter-narrative to psychiatry. And they are going to get excommunicated by their fellow journalists.

BB: So let me ask you: How has it reached this dimension? What is the role of money here? What are the different factors that have come together to make journalists want to drum out anyone who does not tout the party line?

RW: Okay, this is really complicated. Who ends up being assigned as a medical journalist? Sometimes people who worship science. I love science too, by the way. That's why it irritates the crap out of me to see the principles of science being betrayed. Now some reporters are willing to criticize Big Pharma, right? Because that's understood to be a business enterprise. However, they are far less willing to contradict academic psychiatry.

BB: And you see academic psychiatry as the bigger of the two problems?'

RW: Oh absolutely.

BB: We *expec*t Big Pharma to act out of their own financial interests.

RW: Exactly, and academic psychiatrists are supposed to be the storytellers that tell the truth—it's not Big Pharma. And here's a further problem: In order to get into the counter-narrative, you actually have to invest labour. You have to read the sources. And people don't do that. All I can say is, journalism exists within a larger societal narrative, and to go against that conventional narrative which has been sold to us is really hard, and it is isolating. And it is damaging to your career for you end up barred from working in any sort of regular media.

BB: What do we do about that? I mean the media is a huge force in "manufacturing consent".

RW: You know my dream here? I want *Mad in America* to have its own reporters and to become the "go-to place" for covering "mental health".

BB: So that mainstream reporters will turn to you?

RW: Not just that. We will be doing our own reporting. So all I can say, Bonnie, is this: It is not like the media can be converted. It's that you have to create a new media.

BB: I've got you. And you are seeing the social media as a big opportunity to accomplish this?

RW: Yes, last year, for example, we had 1.5 million unique visitors. And now we need to expand this. The problem is we run this on so little money, but if we get a good grant, enough to really run a magazine . . .

BB: God, yes!

RW: Not that this gets around the problem of the mainstream media, which supports the conventional narrative even when seemingly questioning it. You see it all the time. Even as they're supposedly criticizing something, they are embracing it at the same time.

BB: And in the process reinforcing it.

RW: Exactly. I'll give you an example. Did you see this book by Alan Schwarz [2016] on ADHD Nation? It is seen as critical but all is he doing is objecting to the fact that the numbers of kids so diagnosed has gone beyond the 5%. Who's going to disagree that maybe we are diagnosing too many kids when we get up to 13%? And that narrative actually serves to legitimate the diagnosis.

BB: No question, hence my point that reform itself legitimates psychiatry.

RW: Yeah, you know, this is really part of my own evolution. I used to think: Okay, can we just get information about the medications—I left alone the diagnostic part for a very long time. But the root of the problem, of course, is that the diagnostic system is false, and everything flows from that false and corrupted diagnostic system, including efficacy studies. So what you are talking about is tearing down the Tower of Babel, and I think yes, the Tower of Babel needs to be torn down—and the Tower of Babel is a diagnostic system that is invalid and false.

BB: And on that note, let me thank you, Bob, for the important work that you have done and continue to do. And thanks for this engaged and engaging conversation. You know, when I set about this project, I wanted to have the people with whom I entered into dialogue experience a unique sort of interview—one where we are really grapping together with who they are and where truth lies— and I think that's what's unfolded here.

RW: Yes, and you did this. You really pushed me. It is always good to push whoever you are interviewing.

REFERENCES

Schwarz, A. (2016). *ADHD nation*. New York: Scribner.

Whitaker, R. (2002). *Mad in America: Bad science, bad medicine and the enduring mistreatment of the mentally ill*. New York: Perseus Books.

Whitaker, R. (2010). *Anatomy of an epidemic: Magic bullets, psychiatric drugs, and the astonishing rise of mental illness in America*. New York: Broadway Paperback.

Whitaker, R., & Cosgrove, L. (2015). *Psychiatry under the influence: Institutional corruption, social injury, and prescriptions for reform*. New York: Palgrave.

Representative Publications of Robert Whitaker

Whitaker, R. (2001). *Outlook for depression: Has the magic pill approach run its course?* December: Spectrum Life Sciences.

Whitaker, R. (2002). *Mad in America: Bad science, bad medicine and the enduring mistreatment of the mentally ill*. New York: Perseus Books.

Whitaker, R. (2004). The case against antipsychotic drugs: A 50-year record of doing more harm than good. *Medical Hypotheses, 62*, 5–13.

Whitaker, R. (2007). Creating the bipolar child. In S. Olfman (Ed.), *Drugging our children*. Westport: Praeger.

Whitaker, R. (2010a). *Anatomy of an epidemic: Magic bullets, psychiatric drugs, and the astonishing rise of mental illness in America*. New York: Broadway Paperback.

Whitaker, R. (2010b). Weighing the evidence: What science has to say about the prescribing of antipsychotics to children. In S. Olfman (Ed.), *Drugging our children*. Prager: Westport.

Whitaker, R. (2013). Chemical imbalances: The making of a societal delusion. In B. Turner & R. Orange (Eds.), *Specialist journalism*. New York: Routledge.

Whitaker, R. (2017). Psychiatry under the influence. In J. Davies (Ed.), *The sedated society*. New York: Palgrave.

Whitaker, R., & Cosgrove, L. (2015). *Psychiatry under the influence: Institutional corruption, social injury, and prescriptions for reform*. New York: Palgrave.

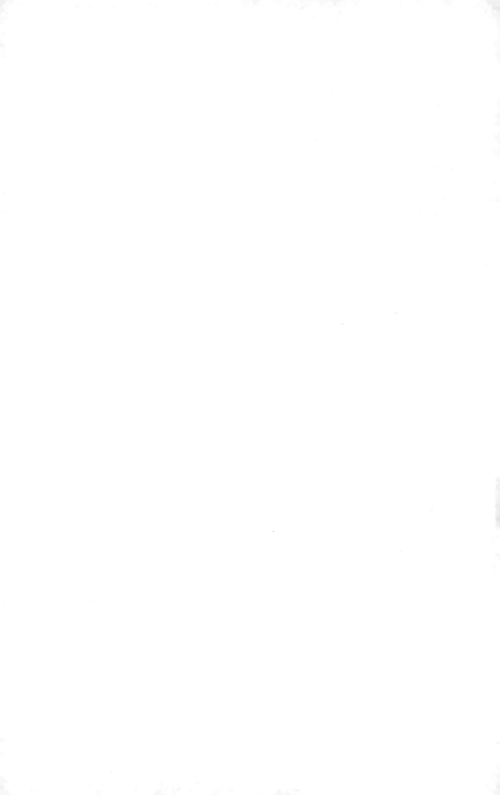

CHAPTER 5

Dialogue with Survivor and Academic Lauren Tenney

Lauren Tenney is a New York psychiatric survivor, an academic, an environmental psychologist, a bad-ass antipsychiatry activist, and the host of a popular blog radio program. She is famous, among other things, for the critical participatory research studies which she has launched. We met each other at the historical PsychOut Conference in Toronto—an international conference centered on resistance to psychiatry which I chaired and which she attended in 2010 (see https://coalitionagainstpsychiatricassault.wordpress.com/events/past-events/psychout-a-conference-for-organizing-resistance-against-psychiatry/). We have been close allies ever since.

BB: It's nice to be talking to you. We haven't talked in so long.
LT: Yeah, really good to hear your voice again.
BB: If you have anything that you are particularly interested in discussing, bring it up at any time. So Lauren, I know that you identify to some degree as part of both the mad movement and the antipsychiatry movement and you mean something slightly different by "mad" than others in the movement do. Why don't we start here?
LT: To be clear, I'm just fine with how others situate themselves in the mad movement; nor overall is there anything which they do that I oppose. Also, let me say that there is far less uniformity here than people think. For example, the US mad movement differs from the mad movement in the rest of the world. And even from one

© The Author(s) 2019
B. Burstow, *The Revolt Against Psychiatry,*
https://doi.org/10.1007/978-3-030-23331-0_5

69

micro-location to another, what is identified as mad varies. Anyway, when I personally talk about mad, what I am talking about is the "righteous rage" type of mad. Also, I think in terms of a link with nineteenth century madness movement—this, because of the Opal. The Opal was a psychiatric inmate edited journal that was a monthly—it was actually part of the income of a New York state lunatic asylum, and indeed was included in their budget in different years. Ten volumes of it were published from 1851 to 1860. More generally, I relate to The Lunatics Liberations Movement in the 1800s. And the Opalians were the inmates who wrote the Opal.

BB: And how does your concept of mad connect up with Opal?

LT: The reclaiming of history, together with words like "mad".

BB: So were the inmates actually reclaiming the word "mad"?

LT: No, but this is what it connects with in my own mind.

BB: Appropriate, for clearly, they *were* reclaiming the word "lunatic".

LT: Yes. What they were up against is concepts like "lunatic", "mad", "insanity". Dementia Praecox [original term for what was later called "schizophrenia"] wasn't on the scene yet—1851–1860. Anyway, to get back to your question, personally, I don't exactly identify as part of the mad movement. I mostly identify as a psychiatric survivor. With the mad movement, it's complicated because many people who so identify simply don't reject psychiatry.

BB: So you're more comfortable with the antipsychiatry movement?

LT: More comfortable by far. At the same time, I'm uneasy with talking about this because...Well...

BB: You maybe feel like you're betraying people?

LT: At times, yes, and I don't want to do that.

BB: Of course not. And it's tricky, isn't it? When identity politics get mixed in with broader politics, and when the identities involved are at once so different and so personal to people, and when, to boot, the analysis which people hold differs, it can be hard to navigate.

LT: Very hard. And you know, there is a huge difference between me and most others. And given my rejection of psychiatry and state involvement, I often get kicked out of mad Facebook groups, though I try to remove myself before that happens. It is especially hard *now* with so many members glorifying psychiatry. When someone challenges the existence of a disorder in a Facebook group, I have seen people literally turn to the moderator and say, "This person is hurting me."

5 DIALOGUE WITH SURVIVOR AND ACADEMIC LAUREN TENNEY 71

BB: It was easier 20 years ago, wasn't it? I mean, because there was far more commonality.

LT: Oh God, was it easier!

BB: Why don't we talk about that? It's hard when a movement is not currently in its heyday and when analyses which were once widely accepted have largely dropped out, which seems to be a truth right now about large parts of the American survivor movement. Now paradoxically, antipsychiatry is once again on the rise, but little of it appears to have penetrated the mad movement. Actually, a development that I particularly notice is the almost complete disappearance of a feminist analysis. Take, for example, what is posted on *Mad in America*. There's seldom a hint of feminism.

LT: Yes, I've noticed that. Since you raised it, to zero in on *Mad in America*, though many good things are attempted there, I honestly don't think that *Mad in America* is "our space".

BB: As in not "movement space"?

LT: Precisely. Now Bob [Whitaker] has done a tremendous job with a lot of things that he never remotely had to do. He has created these exceptional venues—and what he's done is nothing short of phenomenal. But I have very different view from how matters in *Mad in America* are framed and what predominates there. I haven't written for them since the Psychiatric Tsunami piece where I was trying to clarify the enormous state expansion of psychiatric power that was coming down under the Obama administration [see Tenney 2016].

BB: So what does it mean when one venue that for sure falls short of being radical more or less becomes identified as the voice of critique, even, to a degree, the voice of protest? You know, I was part of a group which looked for potential new members almost exclusively via *Mad in America*, which on many levels, struck me at the time and strikes me now as sadly misguided, as important as the website is. For it is treating *Mad in America* as if it were the world.

LT: Actually, my own sense is that the fixation on *Mad in America* spells danger, for they have taken out everything fundamental to our movement. And again, I am uneasy saying what I'm saying, for my critique is not about the people.

BB: Your objections aren't personal, and I surely do get that. And yes, I do see what's been lost. If we look at actual movement publications like *Madness Network News* [an early US movement magazine;

see https://books.google.ca/books/about/Madness_Network_ News_Volume_1.html?id=pQLIBAAAQBAJ&redir_esc=y] or *Phoenix Rising* [an early Canadian movement magazine; see http://www.psychiatricsurvivorarchives.com/phoenix.html], the space was ours, and there was a politic there that was very radical. Which is because they were solidly movement vehicles, whereas MIA [Mad in America] is not, nor is it intended to be but rather is a place for general discussion by critical people, whether they be professionals or survivors. But yes, MIA has more or less assumed center stage, with this becoming the primary location where survivors go. Now *Madness Network News* was not antipsychiatry. Nonetheless, it was hard-hitting, as opposed to something at least partially crafted so as not to alienate progressive professionals, which surely is an inescapable truth about MIA, despite how phenomenal it is. Something, I suspect, that inevitably happens when survivors and the plight of survivors do not have the upper hand. As much as projects may be crafted by people who care about survivors deeply, if oppression is not central, if the analysis is not radical, and if there is not unqualified commitment to getting rid of that oppression and an unflinching grappling with what that entails, and if in addition, irrespective of intention, it ends up occupying the space which once movement vehicles occupied, yes, willy-nilly, a problem exists for the movement.

LT: Also, more generally, I think that the social media dramatically alters the course of everything that we in the movement try to do.

BB: In good ways or bad?

LT: (laughing) Depends on what day it is.

BB: (laughing) Obviously we've got the "Talk with Tenney" Show [see http://www.blogtalkradio.com/talkwithtenney] from social media, which is a positive—and we can talk about that later—but are there negatives as well? Absolutely! In most social media venues, critique is watered down.

LT: And the presence of social media has greatly complicated the movement. Let me zero in on New York, for I know it best. In pre-social media days, you did what you did on a day-by-day basis and then on roughly, a quarterly basis, you got together with others, perhaps made some decisions together, then you returned to whatever it is you were doing.

BB: And by contrast, with social media, people are just posting all the time and are not responsible to anyone—is that the point that you are making?

LT: Yes, but it is beyond that. Think of it like this: With huge numbers of different people one way or another getting connected via the medium, what you have is no longer like-minded individuals getting together. You know, there are over 300 people on my Facebook page right now. And what results from this is conflict. Also cross purposes. The point is, while I am trying to organize activism, others are using these venues largely as a place of mutual support. And these very different purposes really don't work well together.

BB: So the political gets jeopardized?

LT: Actually, as I see it, the political that once so infused the space is long gone. Also, something else we are seeing with social media is how an entire movement or initiative can be dismantled by a single incident.

BB: Let me summarize what I think you are saying: So an incident happens, and everyone hears about it, often hears unfair versions, which in turn, hurts the movement, for thousands of people pick up the message and spread it. Is this what you are getting at?

LT: To a degree, and it is also a question of personal attacks.

BB: Yes, I've seen that. I've seen long term and hard-working members of the movement being totally dismissed because of a difference of opinion that had surfaced on another social media venue. That type of dynamic would not have happened so easily before the social media era.

LT: It complicates things—and not in a good way. It creates distractions. Also, I sense the presence of "plants" in some of the groups.

BB: You are referring to infiltration? Something made easy to do with the huge numbers and the relative anonymity of social media?

LT: Yes.

BB: How about with *closed* social media groups?

LT: It happens there too. And with a group with which I was involved and which was formed to combat the proposed Murphy legislation [psychiatric-power expanding legislation that among things ushered in national outpatient commitment standards], we experience another type of nightmare. Internet administrators actually shut the group down a month before the legislation went before the Senate, at a time, note, when we urgently needed to be talking together and organizing.

74 B. BURSTOW

BB: Ah, yes. Yet another indicator that that the Internet is not exactly a bastion of free speech, for clearly there is behind-the-scenes control. By the way, what reason did they give for shutting you down?

LT: Nothing. They just say: We've decided that this isn't working any more.

BB: So there is an illusion of freedom and self-regulation, when in fact there are administrators with power overlooking you who can shut you down at any minute?

LT: Right. And Facebook has shut me down personally.

BB: A serious problem. At the same time, to turn to the other side of the Internet story, you are one of the people who has made substantial and tremendous use of social media and one of the ways you've done it is by taking up blog radio. Would you like to comment on your use of blog radio?

LT: It's really been great. I am actually in the process right now of putting together a 13-week series on prison psychiatry. And you know, I was able to hook up recently with a regular community radio station here in Albany and clips from the show are going to run on the station. And what I am looking for are people who have been psychiatrized in prison who might be interested in doing their own shows. And through the station, I am actually going to be able to train them.

BB: What a terrific piece of movement building!

LT: Thanks. Anyway, I have been doing blog radio now for four years.

BB: Which is wonderful. And the radio is a great medium for political work.

LT: It is. And I have been able to mount shows where people's voices are really heard. You know, when I think about it, so much has happened since the demise of (de)Voiced—actually, I've never talked about this before—it's been years since I shut down (de)Voiced. And I have had to literally reinvent myself again on how to educate, organize, and focus. That said, one major outcome of (de)Voiced is that people were silenced and retaliated against [for information on the (de)Voiced project, see http://www.laurentenney.us/devoiced.html].

BB: My guess is that we are losing the reader here. Could you explain what (de)Voiced was?

LT: A project which I conducted for my PhD in environmental psychology. I officially started working on it in 2008. It was an environmental community-based participatory action research project. Thirty-six people were involved in its design, all with psychiatric histories.

BB: And what was done that made this "participatory" research?

LT: There were several stages. The first was discussing what my dissertation should be about, what materials I should be reading.

BB: So consultation was involved, but what in particular made this a piece of community participatory action research?

LT: Well, we had six study coordinators by the time it well under way.

BB: And were people taking action?

LT: We put together some videos.

BB: Educational videos for the public?

LT: Right. And we travelled the country interviewing people, helping them tell their "environmental autoworkographies". For this, we used an aspect of environmental studies called "environmental autobiography", where you tell the story of your life with reference to the various environments that you have been in. Not only physical but also social and cultural, religious, spiritual, whatever.

BB: Interesting work. And did this project have a life beyond the thesis?

LT: Not exactly. It is actually under embargo. I will never share the videos again unless they are conscientiously edited.

BB: I detect an incident here. What happened?

LT: One of the leaders was videotaped on a train in the midst of a racist, misogynist rant against a stranger. And the video was sent to me. To make a long story short, that night I contacted the university ethics committee and said that I was shutting down the research. And it's a shame because there were over a hundred people involved. Moreover, we'd created videos that have nothing to do with this person.

BB: Sorry about what happened. And I can see how the inevitable fallout from that would be disheartening. That said, it is good that you had created videos with no connection with the person at the center of the incident. And those videos, did they continue to be distributed?

LT: Yes. After I graduated, I kept aspects of the research running. In fact, it has just recently been approved through a continuing review by the ethics committee. Now I have not shared any of the materials published through the research since I was informed of the incident. The research was officially closed in 2016, but whatever had been published, remains published. The group Surviving Race took on issues of racism and misogyny in the movement following the incident. And many of us are still trying to expose the institutional and structural discriminations that the movement has replicated.

BB: Good to hear. You know, when I think of your history in the movement, what comes to mind first is that you've taken part in a lot of participatory projects. Is it in such activity that you see the hope for a healthy movement? Where people are researching and taking action together?

LT: To be honest with you, I'm not sure about that any more—damn it, I really don't mean to sound so negative!

BB: This has been a disappointing time for you, and I get that. And I aware of how you personally have been attacked, and I'm so sorry about that. Though Lauren, if we can zero in on what hope you have for the movement, insofar as you do see hope, where does that hope lie?

LT: What I've been doing is trying to get involved in broader movements.

BB: Understood. And what do you see yourself as doing five years from now?

LT: Hopefully something that furthers the evidence of psychiatric fraud.

BB: So you want to continue focusing on research?

LT: Yes.

BB: And to continue using social media?

LT: Yes, despite what I said before, a great benefit of social media is that it is a place where we actually can get coverage.

BB: Indeed. To me too, the beauty of social media is it acts as a conduit for voices that haven't a chance of being heard in mainstream venues.

LT: And that's the thing even with blog radio. If you'd have told me even a few years ago, don't worry, soon you are going to be working with a community radio station, I wouldn't have believed you. So there are places where we can go and create traction. And as a movement, ferreting out and using those places, that's what we have to keep doing. And whatever you end up taking up, a curious process sets in. Often, it works well for a while, and other people start to use it and it is good times. And then it gets changed in

5 DIALOGUE WITH SURVIVOR AND ACADEMIC LAUREN TENNEY 77

unfortunate ways, and so you always have to be on the lookout for the "the next thing", the next way to get your message out. Hence my own trajectory from working inside the state, which I did for four years, to going to school, to finding other venues.

BB: So the trick is, you kept recreating yourself in order to have an effect, right?

LT: Right. And you need to know when to move on for the state keeps coming in, taking over, and sabotaging what you do. That said, I would add that despite my flippant comments on participatory research earlier, it is precisely in working together with others in a participatory way that I think the hope lays. I also want to see us focus more on racism, on intersectionality, and the like. There are serious problems in the movement when it comes to racism and the gross inadequacy of the attention that we afford it. Look at it! In New York City, with the Assertive Action Treatment teams, 18% of the people subjected to involuntary outpatient commitment are white, the rest, people of color [see https://www.facebook.com/photo.php?fbid=10158210385510462&l=79ea5a8379]

And more generally, the heaviest of psychiatric attacks land on people of color. And until this movement becomes reflective of who exactly is being preyed upon by psychiatry, we will be sadly missing the mark.

BB: I agree. In Canada as well, we see the same contradictions. The vast majority of the movement is white. Whereas, with the exception of electroshock, who is singled out for the worst treatment are transparently people of color.

LT: Yeah, and this is a problem that needs to be addressed.

BB: Absolutely. So Lauren, are there other questions that you'd have liked me to ask?

LT: Here's what I am wondering about—and I don't have the answer to this and so I am asking you for input—I'm really concerned about this state push toward early diagnosis and how it is going to play out.

BB: Me too.

LT: With the new legislation that has been enacted [for an article of this, see Tenney 2016], there are going to be mandated psychiatric screenings for everyone in the States across the board.

BB: Which I agree is an absolutely terrifying development and something it is critical to organize against. Now the UN's pronouncements on psychiatry's interference with human rights may be something that we can use as leverage. We are talking after all about massive human rights violations. It's at least a route. We could bring in international law. Also national law, for what is happening here may well be unconstitutional.

LT: Yes, I can see using the law in various ways, but what I am looking at here is more the question of social cultural structure. What's it going to mean to have one or two generations who have no idea whatever what it means not to have a diagnosis?

BB: I get your point. If we lose this fight, do we ever lose! For what would emerge is a profound change in both social and personal identity—and one that cuts across the board.

LT: We have already lost it is what I am saying. The point is that in two generations we are going to have an entire society that has no idea what it means to not have a psychiatric label.

BB: If things continue as they are now, you are absolutely right. Which is precisely why we cannot let society continue on this path.

LT: But Bonnie, it is *already* too late, for it is *already law* in the US.

BB: What you're referring to, I presume, is that it is already law that all children have to be psychiatrically screened [The Murphy Bill, HR2646]?

LT: Yes. Which was passed and is now referred to as The Cures Act.

BB: My sense here is that we've lost the battle—not the war. Fortunately, so far there are no laws quite this bad in Canada or the UK, etc., though alas, we are all plagued with the horror of outpatient committal laws. And awful as it is that they passed such legislation in the first place, bad laws can still be overturned.

LT: There is now an expectation that all children will be evaluated.

BB: There is an expectation, which is awful, but so far, it is not in effect and many children still haven't been diagnosed. Isn't that correct? And of course what you are worried about is that once people start applying the law routinely, what happens in the US could very quickly from go from *many* children being evaluated to *all* children. That of course is the danger, and that threat, of course, is imminent.

LT: Within a year or so, by law, every child will be evaluated.

BB: Which means we need to double and quadruple our efforts at fighting back.

LT: But what I am concerned about is 60 years from now.

5 DIALOGUE WITH SURVIVOR AND ACADEMIC LAUREN TENNEY 79

BB: Me too, and if the world 60 years from now is not to be an obscenity of psychiatric rule, we have to fight back now. If 60 years pass with everything going in this direction, change would be far harder, for you would have more or less no one outside of this mindset. Being assessed and being put on drugs would seem as normal as going to school.

LT: Agreed. So how do you craft the message now so that we can prevent a future like this?

BB: You know, as I think about it, crafting the question in a way that makes use of the 60-year framework, as you have done, may well be a good strategy. How about alerting the public to what America and indeed to the world is to become sixty years hence? If the average person started taking in the danger, because we were putting it in their face, might they not start actively opposing? It could even be tailored to specific audiences like new parents.

LT: Right. But what is getting to me is that the legislation has *already passed*. And so it is *too late*. In the books, for example, every pregnant woman is subject to a psychiatric screening.

BB: Which is horrible, and I understand how discouraging it is for those of you fought long and hard to prevent this draconian legislation from passing. But let me suggest, no, it is not game-over. That said, let me check how far the implementation has gone. Everyone on the books is mandated to get a psychiatric screening. Is everyone *actually* getting a psychiatric screening?

LT: It's beginning to happen [Luckily, the government is incompetent].

BB: So then we need active resistance both popular and legal now. We need to mount a concerted attack on all levels.

LT: Right.

BB: We want to safeguard the future? We need to stay focused. We need to steer clear of defeatism. We need a mass movement against laws and practices like this, against what, after all, constitutes a flagrant human right violation, not to mention something that profoundly jeopardizes posterity. And I can see getting traction. Look at the entry into the schools. The penetration of psychiatry into our schools currently is not something that the average citizen exactly wants.

LT: But they've been in the schools for decades.

BB: Indeed, they have been, but I still don't think it is what the average citizen wants. When parents found themselves charged in the US for refusing to have their kids psychiatrically examined, the average person who learned about it was shocked. The point is, we have leverage here. We have intrusion that the average citizen is uncomfortable with. If we use the leverage now and use it focally and strategically, what the world looks like sixty years hence could be very different place from the scenario currently unfolding. So, it is a very good focus. The point is, just as I think that focusing on the attack on children is essential if we wish to safeguard posterity, I likewise think it is good strategy for my sense is that the average citizen is not onside with this government intrusion—they don't want it. And so if we focused 90% of our resistance on what is happening with children, we might in fact be able to pull off a huge reversal.

LT: I am particularly worried about what these new laws are ushering in in the US.

BB: Absolutely. And what happens in the US is pivotal. And once something happens in the US, it happens to various degrees everywhere else.

LT: Yes.

BB: On a related note, I've had an article accepted in a refereed journal, which I wanted to alert you to, called "The Psychiatric Drugging of Children and Youth as a Form of Child Abuse—Not a Radical Proposition" [the article is now out; see Burstow 2017 in the reference section].

LT: Oh that's wonderful news!

BB: It's part of the type of work that I see as necessary to prevent your sixty years hence scenario from materializing. That said, I think all of us in the movement feel the danger you are seeing. Children—this is a particular pivotal area where the psychiatric lobby is winning, where they are creating "repeat customers", where they are destroying lives before they even begin. And this is the number one fight that we need to take on. For indeed, if we let them destroy our youth, that is the future generation. So Lauren, as a starting point, how about if we look toward having an international conference with a total focus on the appalling intrusion on children and what we can do about it. That might well hit the mainstream press. And that might well keep us on track. If we made it extensive enough, we could even use the international conference as an opportunity to begin to create world-wide structures through which we could organize.

LT: Yeah.

BB: Let's do it, Lauren. It calls out to be done. And it is a strategic enough focus that it would bring in people from all sorts of areas that normally would not think of opposing psychiatry.

LT: It's true.

BB: Besides survivors, including, I would add, child survivors, there are social workers. There are parents. There are grandparents. There are lawyers. There are teachers who are beginning to get antsy about what they are being sucked into.

LT: That's right.

BB: So let's capitalize on that. Let's mount a conference intended to kick-start a massive campaign of organized resistance. And let's keep parents focal. The point is, a high percentage of parents don't like what is happening to their kids, don't like this intrusion into their family. And if parents can be mobilized, if they actually take center-stage, who do you think the public will side with? They'll side with parents over professionals. And so that's where I think our biggest push should come from. So, yes, let's do an international conference.

LT: Fabulous! That's really exciting. I'm in. Let me know what I can do to help make this happen.

BB: Indeed, I will. Which is as good a note as any on which to end this conversation. Lauren, thank you for talking with me today.

LT: And Bonnie, thank you so much for including me in this book.

References

ACT Team Data. https://www.facebook.com/photo.php?fbid=10158210385510462&l=79ea5a8379.

Burstow, B. (2017). The psychiatric drugging of children as a form of child abuse—Not a radical proposition. *Journal of Ethical Human Psychology and Psychiatry, 5*(1), 65–76.

Mad in America. www.madinamerica.com.

Phoenix Rising. [an early Canadian movement magazine]; see http://www.psychiatricsurvivorarchives.com/phoenix.html

82   B. BURSTOW

Tenney, L. (2016). *A psychiatric tsunami is upon us.* Downloaded August 30, 2017 from https://www.madinamerica.com/2016/11/warning-psychiatric-tsunami-upon-u-s/

REPRESENTATIVE PUBLICATIONS OF LAUREN TENNEY

Downing, M., & Tenney, L. (Eds.). (2008). *Video vision: Changing the culture of social science research.* Cambridge: Cambridge University Press.

Masel, E. R., & Tenney, L. (2016, March 13). Lauren Tenney on mad activism. On the future of mental health series. *Psychology Today.* Downloaded August 13, 2018 from https://www.psychologytoday.com/us/blog/rethinking-mental-health/201603/lauren-tenney-mad-activism

Tenney, L. (2000). It has to be about choice. *Journal of Clinical Psychology, 56*(11), 1433–1445.

Tenney, L. (2006). Who fancies to have a revolution here?: The opal revised (1851–1860). *Journal of Radical Psychology,* Radical Psychology Network, Winter, 5. http://www.radpsynet.org/journal/vol5/Tenney.html

Tenney, L. (2008). Psychiatric slave no more: Parallels to a black liberation psychology. *Journal of Radical Psychology, 7*(1), 2–11.

Tenney, L. (2014). *(de)Voiced: Human rights now: An environmental community-based participatory action research project. Vols. I, II, and III.* Graduate Center, City University of New York, UMI.

Tenney, L. (2015a, November 24). Electroshocking veterans and their fetuses. *Mad in America.* Downloaded August 13, 2018 from https://www.madinamerica.com/2015/11/electroshocking-us-veterans-and-their-fetuses/

Tenney, L. (2015b, December 30). Shock device as safe as eyeglasses? 89 days to say no. *Mad in America.* Downloaded August 13, 2018 from https://www.madinamerica.com/2015/12/shock-device-safe-as-eyeglasses-89-days-to-say-no/

Tenney, L. (2016a, July 31). *Final report of (de)Voiced. An environmental community-based action research project.* Research terminated July 25, 2016. Report electronically submitted, July 31, 2016. Downloaded August 13, 2018 from http://laurentenney.us/files/117279917.pdf

Tenney, L. (2016b). A psychiatric tsunami is upon us. *Mad in America.* Downloaded August 30, 2017 from https://www.madinamerica.com/2016/11/warning-psychiatric-tsunami-upon-u-s/

Tenney, L. (2016c). Spirituality psychiatrized: A participatory planning process. In B. Burstow (Ed.), *Psychiatry interrogated: An institutional ethnography anthology* (pp. 63–80). New York: Palgrave Macmillan.

Tenney, L., & MacCubbin, P. (2008). No one was watching. In M. Downing & L. Tenney (Eds.), *Video vision: Changing the culture of social science research* (pp. 14–79). Cambridge: Cambridge Scholars Publishing.

CHAPTER 6

On Berlin Runaway House: Dialogue with Wichera

Kim Wichera is an antipsychiatry activist, a writer, a non-binary person, and a member of the Berlin Runaway House collective. An intrinsic part of Germany's survivor movement, Berlin Runaway House is a highly supportive and democratic house for homeless people trying to escape psychiatry, where residents make the major decisions and where many of the staff are survivors. I met Kim a short while ago, when they emailed me asking if I would consider shortening a chapter that I had written in one of my books and allowing it to appear in a book called Gegendiagnose II, *which was to be published in Spring 2019 by the publishing house Edition Assemblage. Naturally, I enthusiastically agreed.*

BB: Thank you for agreeing to this dialogue. How about we begin with something dear to your heart? How would you describe Berlin Runaway House?

KW: It's a facility that has existed for over 20 years.

BB: And really it is a house where people can live who are "running away" from psychiatry. Quite something that you pulled this off!

KW: The organization that wanted to open this began working on it in the 1980s. Took years of negotiations.

BB: And my guess is that the leverage which you had came precisely through connecting it with homelessness, right?

© The Author(s) 2019

B. Burstow, *The Revolt Against Psychiatry,*
https://doi.org/10.1007/978-3-030-23331-0_6

83

KW: Yes. The question was whether to go for funding for people with diagnoses or to do it instead via the homeless sector.

BB: And the homeless sector was easier.

KW: Not only that, we weren't obliged in any way to concern ourselves with diagnoses.

BB: Perfect.

KW: And being antipsychiatry, we don't care about diagnoses. The criterion that we do have to pay attention to is that residents must be at least in danger of becoming homeless. Now the funding is tricky. People move in. And then we request funding for them. And they stay usually about six weeks. The state's definition of crisis means it lasts about 6 weeks.

BB: So a very tight definition. Six weeks is a very short time. But you've also had people stay a lot longer, haven't you?

KW: Yeah, even one and a half years.

BB: Terrific. And so while this is defined as a crisis center and the expectation is a short stay, there is a possibility of people staying longer—which is great, because a longer stay allows for more than just getting past the immediate crisis.

KW: Yeah.

BB: Now one of the things that really impresses me about your house is you are openly antipsychiatry. How in the world did you get state funding while being openly antipsychiatry?

KW: (laughter) Oh, gosh!

BB: That wouldn't happen in North America. Or have you been forced to downplay that aspect?

KW: Not exactly. You know, we had substantial support at the beginning. People from the progressive psychiatry movement stood up and insisted that a house like this was necessary.

BB: Gotchya. And so did the government just sort of ignore the fact that you called yourself antipsychiatry?

KW: Yes. But what was also a factor, at the time when people were mobilizing to open this house, a critique of psychiatry was in the air.

BB: A propitious moment in history?

KW: Yeah.

BB: And if I remember correctly, the house was given to you. And the person who initially gave you this house was a man whose son had killed himself more or less as a consequence of being psychiatrized. Hence his passionate interest in this project.

KW: That's right. The son killed himself after being institutionalized.

BB: This I can really relate to. One of most active members of our group Coalition Against Psychiatric Assault [https://coalition-againstpsychiatricassault.wordpress.com/] joined us precisely because her son had killed himself after years of "psychiatric treatment". He couldn't live with the terrible state to which he had been reduced [in this regard, see Chap. 13]. And I cannot help but feel that here is a constituency we should be upfronting, for it is one the public intuitively understands and can relate to. Question: Do you think, as I do, that such parents are a relatively untapped resource that the antipsychiatry movement should be turning to more?

KW: Well, he just gave us the house. You know, if you are a parent supporting your child, there are not a lot of places you can turn to for help.

BB: I totally agree, and that needs to change. At the same time, parents are a credible constituency that can speak out.

KW: True.

BB: And so the question that I am posing is this: As a new direction, what do you think about antipsychiatry creating venues where such parents can speak out?

KW: Yes, that sounds promising to me. Which reminds me, about a decade ago, there was a young trans person who did not identify with their ascribed gender and this person's mother was supportive. But the office for the youth department had the trans kid picked up and brought to a psychiatric institution. What they said is that what the mother was doing was not right. Anyway, the mother spoke out, which resulted in huge public interest and support.

BB: Good to hear. And yes, that speaks to my point. That said, how about trans people and Berlin Runaway House? Do many transgendered people take refuge in your house?

KW: Yes. Because we are open about our transgender politics.

BB: And because there are openly transgendered staff present like yourself?

KW: Yes, and we reserve the second floor of our house exclusively for women and transgendered people.

BB: So you have a commitment to creating a safe space here on the basis of sex and gender, right?

KW: Yeah. For about nine years now.

BB: Terrific.

KW: And actually, we oppose discrimination of any kind. And of course, that includes sanism. You know, this is the only place in Germany where people are allowed to be crazy.

BB: And you do allow people, if this is their inclination, to descend into "craziness", right?

KW: We do. As long as the other people here are not hurt.

BB: Which reminds me of the days of R. D. Laing, the big difference being—and I see this as huge and what you are doing as far better—you don't have as an agenda people descending into their madness. In fact, you don't impose agendas on residents at all, for this house is survivor-led, not staff-led. Rather you allow people to pursue their own agenda, which, significantly, commonly includes choosing to withdraw from psychiatric drugs. You simply have a house enormously respectful of difference. Which in the process makes a space and provides support for folk reaching into parts of themselves where they feel the need to go.

KW: Yes.

BB: A respectful and truly bottom-up approach. To shift topic here, when we were emailing each other, one of things that you said—and to be clear, I agree—is that psychiatry has changed considerably of late. And so we need a new version of antipsychiatry. What are your thoughts on this?

KW: You know, we've all us read the 1970s antipsychiatry literature. Which is fine but psychiatry has changed greatly since then. How to sum it up? I would say that the population which they are targeting is now much broader.

BB: For sure, they are now widening the net. Now they pretty well want *everyone* under the auspices of psychiatry. Once upon a time, you had to obviously stick out as "not the norm". Now even people who are the norm are targeted.

KW: Precisely. And antipsychiatry needs to theorize this.

BB: Which brings me to a related topic. At Runaway House, you have been pursuing publishing projects for several years now. How and why did this come about?

6 ON BERLIN RUNAWAY HOUSE: DIALOGUE WITH WICHERA 87

KW: That's a relatively long story. I started with a political group that others in Berlin are also part of. The issue with which we were wrestling is: How to reconnect the left with issues of psychiatry?

BB: You say "reconnect". So were they strongly connected at one point in Germany?

KW: Well, yes.

BB: And how successful has your attempt at reconnection been? You know, in North America, one problem we have is that while most antipsychiatry people are left-wing, most of the left is fairly hostile to antipsychiatry. So you are experiencing something different in Germany, are you?

KW: Not sure I can generalize, but much of the left is very open to us and very knowledgeable. And what contributes to this, we have done a lot of workshops with them on it.

BB: So people on the left in Germany actually come to antipsychiatry workshops?

KW: Yes. We look at critiques of psychiatry; and we look at feminism, for example; and we look at how we can work together.

BB: Good to hear. By contrast, in the North American movement(s), we have a very hard time reaching the left. The feminist movement, yes, the feminist movement and the antipsychiatry movement have long been strong allies. But to a great extent—certainly not completely—we have lost the left.

KW: We have put considerable work into this. We've traveled around Germany talking to people about the importance of the left critiquing psychiatry.

BB: Terrific.

KW: And we've been doing this for years. What happened is we started to mount various series of workshops. And we started to mount Mad Pride in Berlin. Actually, almost every year, Mad Pride is held in Berlin and Cologne.

BB: Well, Mad Pride happens throughout North America as well, but while the left is part of it, it is not a particularly left-wing phenomenon.

KW: Now there's a difference between our regions because here it is done almost exclusively by left-wing people.

BB: Interesting! So the mad movement, the antipsychiatry movement, and the left really are allied in Germany?

88   B. BURSTOW

KW: Yeah...And it is out of these alliances that we started publishing. We want to publish on antipsychiatry theory as it relates to the movement at this particular point in Germany. The first antipsychiatry book we published was about 344 pages, and it included articles about antiracism.

BB: Good to hear. That said, what do you see as the main difference between antipsychiatry in Germany and antipsychiatry, say, in the US?

KW: I am looking right now at the New York protest against the APA [American Psychiatric Association]. It's way bigger than anything we do. I would say that in Germany, the movement is much weaker.

BB: Because it doesn't take on full scale activism projects?

KW: Yeah. Some people are doing this. But it's rare.

BB: Ah, but demos is one measure only of a strong movement. You are publishing; you are educating; you are nurturing alliances; you are running a house whose services and politics are exceptional—I would hardly call that "weak". That said, let me ask: what is your vision for the future?

KW: Well, right now, we are facing many difficulties, in particular, financial difficulties, because of the severe limitations on funding. You see, our concept is we want a place where people can be without being forced to do anything.

BB: Which is a good part of why what you offer is so good. But what makes it financially harder to do that today than it was, say, ten years ago? Like, is the rate at which they are funding you not as good as it was previously?

KW: Um...No, the difficulty comes more from the fact than we are not allowed to address certain kinds of stuff in our house. For example, we have to have a certain percentage of social workers. And this is tied to the issue of funding. We have to have at least one social worker in the house for every two residents.

BB: And so they don't care who else you employ essentially. But these other employees do not count in the required social worker quota? I got it. So it is the *exclusivity* of the social worker quota that is causing you problems?

KW: Yes. And we find that arbitrary. It is more important that people who work here have the awareness necessary. Whether because they are survivors themselves, or whatever.

BB: Absolutely, which is what makes your center what it is. Especially the propensity to hire survivors. Now technically they let you hire people other than social workers, but it won't count toward your social worker quota?

KW: And the less social workers, the more cutbacks to our funding.

BB: You're obviously in a double bind here.

KW: So we are trying to negotiate with the state department to get another option with respect to funding. Also, we would like other facilities in the house.

BB: So you would like to expand?

KW: Also to have different places for different people. Not only homeless people.

BB: Understood. You don't want to be limited to this one house and model that you started with. And I can surely appreciate this. You have a vision for the future where there are lots of different houses, all with somewhat different mandates.

KW: Precisely.

BB: A really salient vision. To shift direction and to enter the personal, Kim, what brought you personally to work in a place like Runaway House?

KW: I have never been a "psychiatric patient".

BB: So how did you come to see how horrible psychiatry was for people?

KW: As required, I started working in the social services. You have to do one year in the social services and I began doing that.

BB: What program forces you to do one year in the social services?

KW: Well, in Germany at the time, you had a choice between going into the army or doing social service work.

BB: Got it. So it's like conscription, but you had two options? You could choose social service work? Or chose the army? Interesting.

KW: Yes. And I was working in the psychiatric area. And I expected something very different than what I ended up seeing.

BB: Let me hazard what is not exactly a wild guess. Like most people, you were expecting that psychiatry, as an alleged "helping profession", would actually be "helping" people?

KW: Yes. And instead, what I saw is people being treated absolutely atrociously.

BB: So you found yourself wanting to create something better?

KW: Here's what happened: Shocked by what I had seen, as a political person, I started a radio program critiquing psychiatry, and in one of those radio broadcasts, I interviewed someone from Runaway House. And I decided that I wanted to work there. That was 2005—and the rest is history.

BB: You surely did land in a place that needed you. And we are all of us glad you did. That noted, before we wrap up, is there anything else you would like to talk about?

KW: Actually, I have to go now for my team is asking for me.

BB: Ah yes, the pressures of working in a live-in social service house—I know it well! Kim, good luck with the vital work which you are doing. And thank you for this interview.

[To learn more about Runaway House, see: http://www.peter-lehmann-publishing.com/articles/others/iris_eng.htm]

Kim's Added Comment

Some words about my background: I'm not a psychiatric survivor. I came as a child from Poland to Germany. As this predated the fall of the Iron Curtain, we had to stay for about 18 months in a refugee camp. I was subjected to sexual violence when I was about nine years old. I moved away from home when I was 16 and stayed at a youth shelter for two years. I lived openly as a non-binary person. Eventually, though, I had to go see a psychiatrist as I wanted to start taking hormones—and there was no way in Germany to get them legally without getting diagnosed with gender dysphoria. Now, I rejected and still do reject the very idea of asking the state for an acknowledgment of my gender, but I was in a dependent situation for I needed the medical procedure covered. Fortunately, I was lucky enough to find a psychiatrist who didn't make me pretend that I fit into the standard transitioning narrative in order to get what I needed.

Some words about antipsychiatry/psychiatry:

The psychiatric system has changed considerably and antipsychiatry theory has to catch up if our movement is to remain relevant. Some key points here are:

1. Power in the psychiatric system is not any longer *exclusively* built around social control and oppression. We have to find a way to address a psychiatric system that is creating subjectivity and shaping human experience in order to be able to create a current, matching critique.

2. Psychiatric practice is much more diverse nowadays. There is still violence and forced treatment but also prevention and collaborations with psychological institutions. And an antipsychiatry movement that addresses only the oppressive side of the psychiatric system is lacking terms by which to frame and challenge techniques which are subtle and of a disciplinary nature.
3. During the past century, we have witnessed how the psychiatric system has broadened its focus from people it construes as mad, to each and every one of us. The psychiatric system became a part of all our lives with its adoption of psychological techniques that everyone of us is using to manage his/her emotions, to control and to optimize ourselves.

Psychiatry is therefore much more than an institution. It is a whole system, from oppression and violence to self-optimization, from the closed ward to the self-help book and so forth. We can describe this system as a certain technology of power for a certain kind of society (capitalism). In that sense, the mechanisms of the psychiatric system are similar to sexism, racism, and other systems of power, and therefore the theories about racism, ableism, sexism, and so on are the place where we can find the terms to describe how the psychiatric system is working and how to fight against it.

Literature that I See as Helpful

Burstow, B., LeFrançois, B., & Diamond, S. (2014). *Psychiatry disrupted: Theorizing resistance and crafting the (r)evolution.* Montréal: McGill-Queen's University Press.

Castel, F., & Castel, R. (1982). *The psychiatric society.* New York: Columbia University Press.

Miller, P., & Rose, N. (1986). *The power of psychiatry.* New York: Polity Press.

Preciado, P. B. (2013). *Testo junkie. Sex, drugs, and biopolitics in the pharmacopornographic era.* New York: The Feminist Press.

Rose, N. (2009). *Inventing our selves: Psychology, power, and personhood.* Cambridge: Cambridge University Press.

Schmechel, C., Dion, F., Dudek, K., & Roßmöller, M. (2015). *Gegendiagnose: Beiträge zur radikalen kritik an psychologie und psychiatrie.* Berlin: Edition Assemblage.

CHAPTER 7

Toward a Democratic Psychiatry? Dialogue with Ian Parker

Ian Parker is a psychologist who is a leading figure in Britain's critical psychiatry movement as well as an active member of the editorial collective of Asylum Magazine. *He is also a psychoanalyst, a prolific author, a Marxist with a difference, the editor of a psychology series for Routledge, and a critical discourse analyst. He wrote a chapter for a book of mine several years ago, and we have remained close allies ever since.*

BB: I've been looking forward to this interview, Ian. That said, in the interest of bringing us quickly into the nitty-gritty of your position, let me highlight one of the more stunning remarks that you made in *Psychiatry Disrupted* [Burstow, LeFrançois, and Diamond, 2014—a book of mine in which Ian has a chapter]. You say that psychology as a discipline and practice is deeply moral in the "worst" sense of the word. What does that mean to you?

IP: Put it this way—I distinguish between morality on the one hand and ethics on the other—and the two are often confused in the discussion of ethics in psychology. What psychologists usually mean when they talk about ethics is morality. And morality is a system of social rules or moral codes that people are expected to adhere to— and everything will be fine, the reasoning goes, so long as you follow the rules.

© The Author(s) 2019
B. Burstow, *The Revolt Against Psychiatry*,
https://doi.org/10.1007/978-3-030-23331-0_7

93

94   B. BURSTOW

BB: So instead of ethical understanding being accomplishments to be achieved—what to do or not do are just turned into precepts to obey. Is that what you're getting at?

IP: Yes, I see ethics, as opposed to morals, as our ability to reflect on our actions and to take responsibility for our choices. And for me, the core of ethics is a collective process. So ethics is something that involves deliberation and thoughts about what the consequences of an act will be—but deliberation needs to be carried out alongside other people, and indeed, with our being accountable to others. And that process of deliberation and thought is different than morality, which usually closes down thought because morality tells you how to think and act.

BB: Let me interject some background information here for there is an important context to your thoughts. You are talking about what you call the whole psy complex, not just psychology and not just psychiatry, correct?

IP: Yes. Psychiatry, and psychology, and psychotherapy, and all those disciplines predicated on moral injunctions on how to, you know, treat your children appropriately, conduct yourself in school, behave in prison, and so forth. All of that's part of the psy complex.

BB: And you see all these disciplines as embedded in morals as distinct from ethics?

IP: Unfortunately, they're *usually* embedded in the morals system.

BB: Which essentially means you either follow the rules and perhaps convince yourself that this works. Or—and of course this is not the only other option—you don't follow them and you run into royal trouble—ergo, according to the system, the need to bring in a psychiatrist or a psychologist?

IP: (laughing) Yeah, that's right.

BB: And you see that permeating all the psy disciplines, which I understand includes but is not limited to psychology, psychiatry, psychiatric social work, psychotherapy, psychiatric nursing, etc.

IP: Yeah.

BB: That said, to touch back on something that readers might be wondering about, you prioritize collectivity, stating that ethics is only done collectively. But can't collectivity equally be a problem? For example, didn't psychiatrists get together and create all the diagnoses in the DSM? Wasn't that a collective process?

IP: There is a difference between collectivity in institutions where there are power relations and rules that people are expected to follow, on one hand, and the kind of deliberations that I am talking about. What I am talking about is more like what happens in a self-help group or a political meeting, or a demonstration. It's where people think together about how to address new situations—something that they haven't thought about before. And it is connected to action, to questioning systems of authority, systems of power.

BB: And as you see it, the psy disciplines instead reinforce the status quo as dictated by government and industry?

IP: Yes, and operate as a collective force, that is, as an institution that people have to fit into. Moreover, they target individuals as if we were all separate from each other.

BB: And as if the problems people face can more or less be seen as stemming from their own private psyche?

IP: That's right. And it weakens our ability to challenge those roles.

BB: This is a complex and important discussion. That said, to back up a bit so people get a sense of where you're personally coming from, few people ever enter psychology with the understanding that *the social* is a formidable factor in trying to understand how people live, how people *might* live, how lives go awry. Instead, they are attracted to psychology precisely because they themselves prioritize the individual and the internal—for that's how psychology is constructed. Did you go into psychology already aware of this pivotal problem? Or was the awareness of the social construction of individual problems a learning process?

IP: The former. I was already involved in left-wing politics when I went into psychology. In fact, what I found so fascinating is precisely the way that it turns social political phenomena into individual processes. I was intrigued by the way that psychology worked to individualize politics, to turn it into individual responsibility. So one of the reasons that I went into psychology was to find out how psychology works from the inside. I was never signed up as a psychologist.

BB: Now, correct me if I'm wrong, but you did eventually practice, didn't you?

IP: Eventually, but only after I trained as a psychoanalyst.

BB: You know, I have never talked to anyone before for whom that is the case.

IP: (laughing). You know, some of my comrades used to ask, "Why are you going into such a bourgeois discipline?"

BB: (laughter)

IP: And my thinking was: Well, that's exactly the point. I'm going into it to find out how it works.

BB: And am I reaching here, or somewhere along the way, did you start to feel that it could be turned around? And perhaps you particularly thought that *psychology* could be turned around.

IP: I found there were some alternatives. Quite early on there were some writings in radical psychology.

BB: Like radical therapy, feminist therapy, etc.?

IP: Yeah, and debates were happening about method, about, for instance, the difference between laboratory experiments where psychologists do things to people as if they are push-pull mechanisms and qualitative research, which was about interviewing people and going into communities etc. And so I became interested in those alternatives. Now these alternatives—well, in Britain at least—came under the heading of a "turn to language", and then finally, "a turn to discourse".

BB: Interesting. Yeah, the depiction of the turn was fairly different in North America. But yes, I can see what you made of it. And really on a fundamental level, you're are all about deconstructing, right?

IP: Well, I took on some of those ideas and connected them with debates happening in literary theory, in philosophy, in politics— which includes deconstruction and the work of Michel Foucault. And that's where I found—what shall I call it?—a kind of vantage point by which to stay in psychology and to speak critically about it. The important thing to keep in mind about psychology is this: Although the discipline overall is dreadful, there are lots of excellent people in it who are trying to find more humane ways of operating. And I think that the same is even true of parts of psychiatry. Some psychiatrists notice that something's wrong with the discipline and rebel against it.

BB: I agree with you *to a point, though only to a point,* about psychology— I am significantly closer to Roland Chrisjohn here [see Chap. 2]. I can see what you are saying about psychiatry too. Nonetheless, my sense is that it has to be thought of differently. With psychiatry, those who see there is something wrong and thereby shift, are in essence not acting like psychiatrists, not acting like medical doctors at all.

IP: Yes, that's right.

BB: Which is a qualitatively different phenomenon than what happens in psychology. There are realms in psychology not predicated on individualism, which is not to say that on some level, the operant principles are not still problematic. And there are people in psychology—take community psychology—who have always approached psychology as a field which is supposed to be about process and supposed to be communal. By contrast, psychiatry as a field is inescapably predicated on the emotional problems people face being inherently medical. And willy-nilly, the thought that it can be "reformed" ignores that basic reality. Which, incidentally, is part of what worries me about aspects of *Asylum*. I mean the magazine is called *Asylum: Magazine for a Democratic Psychiatry*—and I think the goal implicit in the title is an impossible one, for it ignores the utter faultiness at the base of the discipline. The point is that psychiatry's very raison d'être is a bogus claim to medicine. How can that ever be democratic? And how could that ever be okay?

IP: (laughing). You know, Thomas Szasz was in Britain just before he died. Now someone asked for his autograph—and because there was no piece of paper for him to write it on, they handed him a copy of *Asylum Magazine*. Anyway, Szasz took out his pen as if about to sign. Then he looked at us and said, "I'm not going so sign that—it's got the word 'psychiatry' on it."

BB: My hunch is that you see that as a kind of idiosyncrasy. I don't. You know, whatever Szasz's shortcomings were—and I don't deny he had some whoppers—let me suggest that he was absolutely right that the problems with psychiatry are utterly fundamental and have to be approached as such. Like you can't just add the word "democratic" and stir.

IP: Yes, but for us, you know, this phrase "democratic psychiatry" has a particular resonance. It has a connection with abolition which perhaps it does not have in Canada—note the abolition of the mental hospital in Trieste and the democratic psychiatry movement in 1970s [actions and a movement in Italy spearheaded by psychiatrist Basaglia, which was a radical political movement].

BB: There is no question that it was an amazingly radical political movement and there is no question that it had an abolitionist bent and if orchestrated well, "hypothetically", could be a conceivable route to total abolition. Nonetheless, it did not happen then and it is not happening now. The name, moreover, papers over problems. If you have a psychiatry, which, say, is democratic to the extent that you are not locking people up or treating them against their will, there is *less of* a problem at least for the time being for sure but there is *still* a problem. By holding fast to the discipline, you are defining the ground in a certain way, more explicitly, you are defining it as medicine. Define it that way and to varying degrees, people will still be conned into taking substances that will injure them in the mistaken belief that they are bone fide medicine—and the state will still be paying for it to boot. That's a problem. And that's "democratic psychiatry", so to speak.

IP: What you're saying is interesting. It resonates in some way with the arguments of Szasz, who was against psychiatry as a state welfare system. Szasz argued against both psychiatric coercion and psychiatric excuses. He opposed the way that psychiatry was used as a system of control, but he also opposed state-sponsored psychiatry offering help to people needing places of refuge. He attacked Franco Basaglia, in Trieste, for example, because the alternative to the mental hospital that Basaglia put forward were community mental health centres where people could stay for the night [for information on Basaglia, see https://en.wikipedia.org/wiki/Franco_Basaglia].

BB: To be clear, Szasz was right-wing. I am left-wing. So unlike him and like Basaglia, I want services available—and on a basis of something other than private enterprise. Nonetheless, Szasz's comprehensive critique of psychiatry per se is sound: All of psychiatry is problematic. Correspondingly, the reforms that you are talking about were themselves framed in a way that is problematic. Note, there is nothing *particularly medical* about having a place to stay for the night. Of course such things should be provided, but to tie it to a bogus medical discipline is problematic. And what is even more fundamental, do we really want what is offered to people to be centralized, professionalized, and controlled by the state?

IP: I admit I am being mischievous here. But the thing about democratic psychiatry is that although it is called "psychiatry", it is actually doing something quite different—and it includes a space for people who are antipsychiatry, people who want other kinds of community initiatives.

BB: But why tie it to psychiatry at all? And yes, they are doing better things than mainstream does, but if you tie it to psychiatry and psychiatry continues to have an interest in the maintenance of biological psychiatry—and let's be clear, it has to have for it is psychiatry's only raison d'être—then irrespective of the advances made now, the advances will ultimately dissipate for biological psychiatry will inevitably return with a vengeance. Just look at history here. The turn in psychiatry in the eighteenth century to moral treatment didn't look all that different than what we are seeing now with "democratic psychiatry". It too was less coercive, it was practiced by people who were not doctors as well as by doctors. It was based on social principles like human caring and the importance of community and not on the creation of presumptive biological disorders. And it too included retreats where people could stay. Fine. But the reality is that it changed nothing in the long term for psychiatry remained intact. In the fullness of time, biological psychiatry roared back with a vengeance. And we have seen that cycle repeating itself again and again.

IP: I don't disagree with you for the most part. Maybe what we disagree about is whether we can take the labels and use them in a more radical way so as to unravel them—and I think that this is what "democratic psychiatry" does. It effectively destroys psychiatry from within. And I think it is an opportunity worth seizing and working with.

BB: And part of me would love to think that too. You know, I wrote an article called "Liberal Mental Health Reform—A Fail-Proof Way to Fail" (https://www.madinamerica.com/2014/11/liberal-mental-health-reform-fail-proof-way-fail/). And the point of the article is that however exciting such processes look in the short run, what history tells us is that in the long run, such attempts always fail. My God! Were I around when the moral management revolution set in, I may well have "jumped on the bandwagon". I might have said to myself: This is terrific, they are not "bleeding" people, they are not keeping them in chains, they are talking to them, they are setting up country retreats where people in difficulty with themselves can stay. They even allow non-doctors to head such retreats! But did this lead to the end of psychiatric rule? Of the rule of biological psychiatry? Hardly. A hundred years later, biological psychiatry came roaring back, with psychiatry even more biological than it had been previously.

IP: Yeah.

BB: Why? Because psychiatry was upheld in the process. And Ian, I think we do have to learn from history.

IP: But I don't think that democratic psychiatry as it developed in Trieste and in the way it now inspires Europe's radical mental health movement in Europe operates as a psychiatric institution. This phrase "democratic psychiatry" brings together people who are fundamentally critical psychiatry. It's just one of the avenues that we take in dismantling psychiatry.

BB: But to go back to my example, a high percentage of moral management folk for the longest while also didn't operate like an institution.

IP: Many of the people in the movement in Britain, in the magazine *Asylum*, for example, are as hostile to the psychiatric system as you are.

BB: To be honest, that's not my experience, though I do see your point. And for sure, *Asylum* has done some wonderful things. Nonetheless, besides not being abolitionist, there are aspects of it that strike me as highly liberal.

IP: Yeah, I know, and I have been attacked for that.

BB: (laughter)

IP: My comrades accuse me of being a Menshevik because of my relationship with *Asylum*.

BB: My problem is not with you, who I see as a stellar ally. At the same time, I cringe when I see articles in *Asylum* arguing that psychiatry is not providing enough "services" to people—which position is *the very opposite* of an abolitionist agenda. Yes, I want services for people, but why look to psychiatry for it? And indeed, why professionalize it at all? Which brings me to the issue of words. You know, one of the differences between us as well as one of our similarities is the attention that each of us pays to language. You and I both agree that words are critically important—and part of resistance revolves around words. Now sometimes we can reclaim words. Take the "mad movement" reclaiming the word "mad". But I don't think that you can reclaim a word which an institution as powerful as psychiatry owns. Not "mental health", and more fundamentally still, not "psychiatry".

IP: Yeah, where I agree with you is—neither of us want to make psychiatry into something that still functions, albeit in a more democratic way. And I don't think that's where democratic psychiatry leads. The dynamic of democratic psychiatry is actually to undo psychiatry, to unravel it. You know, most of the people involved are not actually psychiatrists. Think of it this way. It is just a space—a space we seize in order to put forward the arguments. It is not that we work in psychiatric institutions.

BB: Nor did most of the people involved in moral management. And to return to the question of words owned institutionally, insofar as they are intrinsically the property of an institution; they can be yanked back by that institution any time they wish. And beyond that, in their own way, they legitimize the institution.

IP: Yeah, I understand that.

BB: And what goes along with this, I worry about cooptation, the likelihood of which is huge. As for cooptation generally, right now we are witnessing huge co-optation even in the Open Dialogue movement [a "non-coercive" movement based on dialogue that is sweeping Europe and North America]. In some countries, psychiatry has virtually taken over this approach.

IP: We have that problem with Open Dialogue in the UK as well. And you are right; more and more psychiatrists are taking training in it and folding it into psychiatry. And it is functioning like a new opportunity for psychiatry to essentially glue people back into their families.

BB: That's exactly it.

IP: But again, I would say that some people are attracted to the Open Dialogue approach for very good reasons.

BB: Absolutely, but to be clear, it is not the approach I object to but the connection maintained with psychiatry.

IP: It gives people a space to talk. And some of the psychiatrists involved in it are starting to break from the logic of the psychiatric apparatus. You know, much as I dislike psychiatry and psychiatrists, there are some *good* psychiatrists.

BB: And no one is questioning that. Just like there can be good prison guards, etc. In fact the existence of good psychiatrists is an old truth which has never changed the nature of the system. Let me ask you something: except for the credibility which it bestows—credibility which comes at a huge price—what's to be gained by retaining that name? Of course, we all understand practitioners who retain the name for strategic reasons in the here-and-now. I think

Peter Breggin, for example, needs to retain the name psychiatrist for otherwise he would not be able to provide expert testimony in a court of law—something that he does in the service of people hurt by psychiatry. But that's a short-term expedience. Not the ultimate direction in which we need to go. And hardly the name to be bestowed on a revolutionary movement.

IP: At least democratic psychiatry starts to connect the word "democratic" with "psychiatry".

BB: Ah, but you're seeing that as positive whereas I am seeing it as a slippery slope that will inevitably lead to defeat. Actually, you know I am thinking here? The very different positions that the two of us are taking each have a logic to them. The question is, though, which of us is right? And my concern is that when we enter the realm of simplistic reform, we squander the moment for profound change. It neutralizes everything and creates the pretense that we are all in it together—rather than addressing power differences and taking seriously the workings of the system. And insofar as nothing is envisioned or acted upon except improving psychiatry—and that's overwhelmingly what I am seeing—in fact, you are actually just preserving the system.

IP: Let me ask: You are not against reforms, are you?

BB: No, but it critically depends on the direction which the reforms take. And when it comes to psychiatry, I am in favor of only those reforms which lead in the direction of abolition.

IP: Yes, me also.

BB: And not those reforms that help it grow and/or make it more palatable to people, that make it better, finer.

IP: So I guess what we are disagreeing about is the question of strategy.

BB: Yes. I suspect to some extent also the question of state control. Also the actual nature of the players today.

IP: You know, the critical psychiatry network will be involved in the conference on psychiatry that *Asylum* is holding in the fall. And they are psychiatrists.

BB: They are—but again let me suggest that the type of the reform that they are about, parallels what happened with moral treatment.

IP: I think we are doing something different. The critical psychiatry network is enabling the professionals who are starting to break from psychiatry to speak with users of services and with other professionals. And in that way, it has the dynamic of reforming in a direction that you and I want. It reforms and it dismantles psychiatry.

BB: It reforms for sure, but dismantling is very different, and at the moment, I am seeing almost no commitment to dismantle—in fact I am seeing a distinct aversion by many to anyone with an abolitionist agenda. Now, is dismantling one of the logical possibilities? Of course, but it is not likely to happen without the presence of some kind of abolitionist principles—principles which I see no evidence of being seriously entertained in critical psychiatry circles now, unlike in the 1990s when you were part of a group called Psychology Politics Resistance [a left-wing UK activist group out to change the psych disciplines; see Parker 2014]. Any chance of our seeing a resurgence of it?

IA: Well, I hope so, but at the moment I am putting my energy into *Asylum Magazine*.

BB: For the benefit of readers with but a passing familiarity with this important magazine, *Asylum* is a British magazine with a fair-sized readership—with both professionals and survivors critiquing and responding to different aspects of the "mental health system". And it has been going since…

IP: 1986 was the first issue.

BB: And as mentioned earlier, the full name is *Asylum Magazine for Democratic Psychiatry*.

IP: And we see the bringing together of psychiatry and democratic in the name as positive.

BB: Which brings us back to the difference between us. I understand the use of the word "asylum" because you are attempting to reclaim the word.

IP: We are.

BB: Which makes sense to me, because "asylum" originally denoted a place of peace, a place of rest, a refuge. And part of your vision— and I would add, mine also—is that there should be such places, correct?

IP: Yes

BB: And "asylum", I would agree, is a totally salvageable word. "Psychiatry", on the other hand, I would suggest, is an utterly unsalvageable word. So what I see you as having done in the very naming the magazine is link together a word that can be reclaimed with a one that is not amenable to reclaiming.

104   B. BURSTOW

IP: You would say it's not possible to reclaim?

BB: It's possible to reclaim the word "asylum", but no, I am suggesting that it is *not* possible to reclaim the word "psychiatry".

IP: I see.

BB: Let me say a bit more about why I see it this way. Initially, psychiatry, of course literally meant treatment of the soul, which might look promising but the point is that it very quickly came to mean something extremely different. Now I know that the word "mad" has been reclaimed even though it had largely a negative connotation in the past. The difference, however, is that it is a word that was also used highly positively in the past so you *could* reclaim it—note, in this regard, the centuries long concept of "divine madness". By contrast, "psychiatry" officially designated and only designated a certain group of people legally endowed with horrendous power over those seen as mad, together with "expertise" in a field defined and recognized as medical.

IP: Yeah, I agree with everything you are saying. Nonetheless, this is one of the banners that we organize under, and what we're doing with it is quite different from what medical psychiatry does.

BB: For sure, and I do get that.

IP: You know, mainstream psychiatric institutions really dislike democratic psychiatry. They dislike critical psychiatry because it is a critique and as such, is a threat of their power.

BB: Agreed, but I've seen the opposite also. Take the critical psychiatry folk who are actually psychiatrists whose writing we come across in *Asylum*, or for that matter, in *Mad in America*. Now I am in no way suggesting all the MIA critical psychiatrists are like this—but many are transparently leveraging themselves and psychiatry more generally to prevail by joining the reform movement. They are in part strategically embracing reform as a way to protect psychiatry, as a way to safeguard it, which is, indeed, the very opposite of an abolitionist agenda.

IP: Yes.

BB: So, much as I value many of them, "critical" psychiatrists worry me. That said, to return to you personally, you yourself are somebody with a real vision for society and someone clearly committed to fundamental social change. So let me ask you. What are your goals? What, say, is your medium and long term vision?

IP:	(laughing) I'm reluctant to answer that question. The problem is, when we start to think about blueprints for the future, we're always confined by the parameters given by present day ideology. Well, here's a way of answering your question—I do see practices in this system which are points of resistance, and which gives indications of how society might be organized in a more caring, open, inclusive way. I see that in the networks of people who are supporting others who are in the mental health system. I see it in aspects of the left. And you know, I would include in that the feminist networks who provide profound critiques of left organizations, of traditional Marxism, for example, who make the connection between the political and the personal, and who would argue that what we do in our everyday lives is as important as the big political programs that we fight for.
BB:	Yes, and I think that you are absolutely right about the enormous importance of this.
IP:	And so when it comes to social change, yeah, I'm a Marxist but I'm a Marxist interested in—I'm not sure how to put this….
BB:	In everyday life?
IP:	In everyday life, yes, which I think all Marxists should be and the best Marxists have been.
BB:	For sure how we operate on an everyday basis could not be more important. At the same time, we have a system that we need to dismantle. And while part of this can happen through erosion, I also think we need to investigate systemic ways of how to bring various systems down. And here, I think, concrete vision and even goals to a degree have a role to play. Dialogue, you and I agree, is enormously critical. So too, though, I would suggest, are strategic goals. Am I right that we disagree on that?
IP:	We agree so far.
BB:	You know, I teach a course called "Creative Empowerment with the Disenfranchised", which is all about working in alliance with the social movements of disenfranchized populations, and in this course the types of questions that we ask ourselves are: What does strategic resistance look like? What do people want? And what of that can we help them get? And how?
IP:	Well, I'm fine with that, yeah. And I think that's in line with the best practices of left politics—that you try and build something as groups and organizations with alternatives to the dominant ones.

You try to build a better society. Which is why the notion of the psych complex is so important. Because it takes you beyond psychiatry as such. It helps you look at the way that psychiatry is embedded within broader networks of institutions and power relations and it helps you see how psychological and psychiatric ideas are used in those institutions to divide people, to prevent people from working collectively together. And it shows the importance of change happening not only in and against the psychiatric system but also, as you have said, in the schools, and so on. I mean there is the whole question about the organization of knowledge here and the expertise that is conferred on professionals, when instead we should be experimenting together.

BB: We need strategic resistance; we need de-professionalization; and we also need experiments that prefigure the society that we are trying to create. And here once again, in important ways, you and I agree.

IP: Even while disagreeing?

BB: Precisely. As a final observation, let me just add that I think that all of us radicals in the "professions" are to varying degrees in a strangely seductive and at the same times untenable position. We get to be experts and anti-experts at the same time—we get, as it were, to "have our cake and eat it too"—but only insofar as our revolts are not fully successful. A complicated contradiction to navigate ethically, wouldn't you say?

IP: Interesting.

BB: And on that note, Ian, thank you for consenting to this interview. And thanks for your part in allowing this to develop into an honest and hard-hitting conversation.

Reference

Parker, I. (2014). Psychology politics resistance: Theoretical practice in Manchester. In B. Burstow, B. LeFrançois, & S. Diamond (Eds.), *Psychiatry disrupted* (pp. 52–74). Montreal: McGill University Press.

Representative Publications by Ian Parker

Parker, I. (Ed.). (1999). *Deconstructing psychotherapy*. London: Sage.

Parker, I. (2014a). Psychology politics resistance: Theoretical practice in Manchester. In B. Burstow, B. LeFrançois, & S. Diamond (Eds.), *Psychiatry disrupted* (pp. 52–74). Montreal: McGill University Press.

Parker, I. (2014b). Madness and justice, *Journal of Theoretical and Philosophical Psychology, 34* (1), 28–40.

Parker, I. (2014c). It's the stupid relationship. In D. Loewenthal & A. Samuels (Eds.), *Relational psychotherapy, psychoanalysis and counselling* (pp. 130–139). London/New York: Routledge.

Parker, I. (2015). Towards critical psychotherapy and counselling: What we can learn from critical psychology (and political economy)? In D. Loewenthal (Ed.), *Critical psychotherapy, psychoanalysis and counselling: Implications for practice* (pp. 41–52). London: Palgrave.

Parker, I. (2017). Marxist theory and psychotherapy. In B. M. Z. Cohen (Ed.), *Routledge handbook of critical mental health* (pp. 244–250). London/New York: Routledge.

Parker, I. (2018). *Psy-complex in question: Critical review in psychology, psychoanalysis and social theory.* Winchester/Washington, DC: Zero Books.

Parker, I., Georgaca, E., Harper, D., McLaughlin, T., & Stowell-Smith, M. (1995). *Deconstructing psychopathology.* London: Sage.

CHAPTER 8

"Activism Is My Real Job": The Mad Movement in Chile Dialogue with Tatiana Castillo

Hailing from Chile, Tatiana Castillo is an antipsychiatry and mad movement activist—and an ally to survivors. For the past few years, along with other Chilean activists, she has been a critical part of the awakening of the mad movement in Chile. I first came across Tatiana and her work about a year ago. I instantly appreciated both what her groups were doing and her own personal commitment.

BB: Nice to be speaking with you, Tatiana. Could you say something about what your role is in the current mad movement in Chile and how you personally became involved?

TC: My role is as an ally and activist. Those of us who do not consider ourselves mad identify as allies.

BB: And you're not paid for working in this area?

TC: Exactly.

BB: So you're doing it solely out of political commitment. And you're an enormously active member of a number of key organizations. Like Cátedra Libre Franco Basaglia and Autogestión Libre-Mente? How did you get involved?

TC: While studying anthropology, I became interested in "mental health". And at that time, I knew nothing about the survivor or the antipsychiatry movement. But as I learnt about it, I grew progressively more drawn to it. I remember encountering one of the active collectives [Center for Critical Action in Mental Health] who

© The Author(s) 2019   109
B. Burstow, *The Revolt Against Psychiatry*,
https://doi.org/10.1007/978-3-030-23331-0_8

presented on their work. And before I knew it, I was following them on Facebook and attending their events. Which is primarily where I learnt about the antipsychiatry movement.

BB: You know, you mentioned antipsychiatry twice now. Now I very consciously identify as antipsychiatry, but my sense is that in Chile, the vast majority of you identify rather as part of the mad movement. But you personally identify with both. Is that correct?

TC: Exactly. And when you talk about antipsychiatry, this often scares "users" of the mental health system. They think people are against them for taking psychiatric drugs.

BB: Yes, I've seen that here as well.

TC: So we tend to avoid the term. Nonetheless, much of what we do is actually antipsychiatry activism.

BB: Now I personally am very excited by what you Chilean activists are doing. You know, most of the movement people in the rest of the world who don't define themselves as antipsychiatry somehow entangle themselves in the state, whereas the Chilean groups have very rigorously steered clear of the state. As far as I can see, you're a genuinely participatory movement, and beyond that, an anarchist movement. You routinely use anarchist conceptions and words like "collective", "gathering", and what is still more telling "prefigurative". Is this purposeful on your part?

TC: Some of us are consciously and purposely framing the movement this way. Others, no. It is similar in this regard to what happens with antipsychiatry.

BB: Are you saying, what movement people do in Chile is largely anarchist, even though they don't use the concept?

TC: Exactly.

BB: Now it is clear that some of your writers are highly familiar with the phenomenon. No one uses words like "prefigurative" by accident. And a central group of which you are a part—Autogestión Libre-Mente [translation: Self-Managed Free Mind]—actually holds its meetings in an anarchist center. Moreover, you very clearly define yourself as critiquing not only psychiatry but the neoliberal state.

TC: Exactly. We don't just want to *change* the "mental health system". We want to *eliminate* it. More generally, we're out to change society.

BB: I can see that. So you're intrinsically a revolutionary movement?

TC: Yes, we are about overall societal change.

BB: What an exciting development! My sense is that in Chile, you are actually leading the way right now.

TC: I think we are.

BB: You are genuinely participatory. You are working for fundamental social change. And you consistently point out that the real experts are not the professionals. They are rather the people with the "lived experience".

TC: Exactly. And here's something that I find really interesting for it shows what sets us apart. One of our members attended a meeting in Ireland for survivors and was very disappointed in what saw there. He saw groups embedded in the system, who received considerable financial support from the state. And when he got up on stage and began talking about what we in Chile do, how everything is self-managed, how we steer clear of system and state funding, the survivors from Ireland were utterly surprised. They exclaimed, "but how can you guys do all those activities with no money?" But it *is* possible. The reality is that we don't need financial support from any institutions. We do it by ourselves.

BB: Yes, and when you do it by yourselves, you are at once acting out of and creating community. And you are in no way an extension of the system.

TC: Exactly, and we don't have to change our words or our message for anyone. We can say whatever we want.

BB: To zero in on some of the central organizations in your movement, a particularly formidable one is called "Cátedra Libre Franco Basaglia" [translation: Free Lectures Franco Basaglia: for its Facebook page, see https://touch.facebook.com/CLFrancoBasaglia/?__tn__=C-R]. I take this is primarily an academic space.

TC: It is. And in that particular group, we primarily operate in a university context.

BB: And as grass roots activists, has that connection with the universities ever posed problems for you?

TC: It very much has at times. It is difficult for us to acquire spaces for free, and universities help us a lot with that. But now they can want to put their stamp on our events and to have some say over what we do. However, that's something we're not open to. We are a grass roots movement after all. And sometimes, we've had to respond: No, we don't want your name attached to our activity events.

BB: I get it. You're protecting your grass roots and radical nature.

112   B. BURSTOW

TC: And we don't want anyone to change any part of what we are doing. So if we want to say antipsychiatry, then we have to feel free to say it. A lot of institutions don't like that. Now sometimes, there is excellent support for what we are doing. And at other times, academics, for instance, will complain about what we're doing. Mostly, though, they've allowed us to speak from our own political perspective.

BB: Good. Now I've noticed that over the last few years you guys have taken a very strong stand on electroshock. Was that inspired by the international protest against electroshock that happens on or just before Mother's Day?

TC: It was.

BB: You know, in Toronto, we initially kickstarted that international protest about 15 years ago. And we decided to situate it on or just before Mother's Day, using the slogan "Stop Shocking Our Mothers and Grandmothers".

TC: I suspect that's because electroshock is very much a feminist issue.

BB: Precisely. That noted, while we are on the question of feminism, let me say that one of the things that has happened in North America is that while we began with a very strong feminist analysis, over the years, it has largely disappeared. If you go on *Mad in America*, for example, you seldom see a single article that integrates feminism.

TC: That's true.

BB: So what has the Chilean movement been doing with respect to feminism?

TC: One of our groups—and it is an offshoot of the larger group Autogestión Libre-Mente—is a space where mad women specifically reflect on their situation. The group's called "It Is Not the Same to Be a Mad Woman as a Mad Man". Both mad women and women allies belong to this group. And they put on many events and make many presentations. And as result, the larger feminist movement has started becoming interested.

BB: Great. You know, I can't believe how much you guys have accomplished in the last few years! Very little was happening. And suddenly you were a major force, pulling off incredible avant-garde initiatives. And throughout you have remained clear about who the real experts are. And that distinguishes you from most other parts of the movement, including in the rest of Latin America, even Brazil and Argentina.

TC: There is not really a survivor movement in those countries. It's important to point out that the movement in Latin America is centered in the fight against the asylum—and somehow they just ignore the use of drugs.

BB: So it's nice to see the centrality of survivors in your movement, also to see you referring to "experts through experience". It is likewise good to see your use of the concept "prefiguring". What you are really saying is, "In how we operate now, let's build in the type of society we are trying to create."

TC: Yes. Now my sense is that antipsychiatry has largely died out in the rest of the world. As a leader in the antipsychiatry movement, what do you think?

BB: For decades antipsychiatry was more or less "dead in the water"—that is, everywhere except Toronto. But in the last five or six years, the situation has changed astronomically. You know, when I first was asked to blog for *Mad in America*, one of the people in charge requested that I not use the word "antipsychiatry".

TC: Wow!

BB: So I refrained—but for my first blog article only. After that I systematically used the word, and progressively, what I found is that there was once again an audience to whom that word spoke.

TC: Yes, but I noticed that you've also had a lot of opposition to your antipsychiatry scholarship.

BB: Let me put it this way: There was opposition sure, but there was also support. And you know, opposition does not worry me. It is an opportunity to educate. Now there are others in our related movements who have a watered-down position in part because they do not want to alienate professionals. The thing is, though, given this modus operandi, it is dubious how far they are going to change the world.

TC: And that's what I see the critical psychiatry as opposed to the antipsychiatry movement is doing. And you know, the bias toward professionals inherent in all this, we have seen this here as well. When survivors have spoken out about how professionals have abused them, the professionals in our midst often get really offended. Not unlike what happens when feminists criticize men and men become threatened.

BB: It is hard for professionals to take in that we need *less* professionals, *not more*, and we need ones that take direction from the average

	human being. And insofar as they have valuable skills, the professionals need to work at transferring those skills to the community.
TC:	And I've noticed it is really difficult for most professionals to reflect in a hard-hitting critical way about their profession.
BB:	Yes, they have a vested interest in taking the position that despite reform being needed, and perhaps even urgently, "mental health professions" have an inherent legitimacy. And it is easy for quasi-progressive professionals to take comfort in the fact that they are simply better than the majority of their colleagues. But obviously, that's not good enough.
TC:	Exactly.
BB:	The point is, they are still pathologizing, and they are still acting as if professionals should be able to exercise control over people's lives.
TC:	And in Chile—and I suspect in other parts of the world—though it is important to do it—it is complicated bringing together survivors and professionals because when you get down to the nitty-gritty, a high percentage of the professionals don't want to hear what survivors have to say.
BB:	Nonetheless, you have created a large number of gatherings in which the two constituencies are brought together. Have you seen professionals take in the problem at a deeper level?
TC:	We have, but mostly in the case of students who are still in the process of forming their identity.
BB:	Yes. Students are one of our hopes. And instead of succumbing to cooptation or to institutional perspectives, a minority end up working at de-professionalizing their profession. At which point, they become a force for transformation.
TC:	Now something interesting has happened here. There was a moment when many students participated, especially in our weekly meetings. But the problem was that it was really difficult for them to remain quiet at times. A lot of them had a critical perspective but it was not enough to understand the centrality that had to be given to survivors. And they often felt left out because no one was asking for their "professional opinion".
BB:	I get it. And a variant of this problem exists even with legendary trailblazers—for they remain at least to an extent, a product of institutional-think. You know, when I look at the legendary work of the professional after whom your organization Cátedra Libre

Franco Basaglia is named, while I greatly admire much of what Basaglia did, at the same time, I am aware that his was a top-down movement, this despite the use of words like "democratic". It was engineered by a psychiatrist and with a psychiatrist left in charge. Do you have a critique of that as well?

TC: We do, because he was first and foremost a professional.

BB: Yes, and he was in essence putting professionals in charge of these "non-asylum" asylums.

TC: Yes. What we like is his legacy of closing down the asylums. However, we are aware that the asylum logic remained.

BB: It surely has. And one of the things I admire about your work in Chile is that you have remained acutely aware of the persistence of asylum logic even when people are being quote-unquote "progressive".

TC: You know, in Chile, it is considered progressive to talk about "community mental health" but in reality, it is not.

BB: Because community mental health essentially remains the asylum in a new garb?

TC: Yes. Now communicating with the professional community, while important, is not our primary interest. We more want to reach the user community.

BB: And at the same time, you are trying to reach society at large, right?

TC: Exactly.

BB: Which makes you a genuine revolutionary movement. Question: Have the movements in other Latin American countries like Argentina and Brazil started to turn to you for guidance?

TC: To some degree, principally through Facebook. For instance, through our page "Mad for Our Rights". And we are starting to see self-help groups form in these other countries.

BB: Terrific.

TC: It is. Nonetheless, I believe our work is looked at uneasily by professionals who lead movements in other Latin American countries.

BB: What a shame! And what do you see on the horizon for the Chilean movement in the next, say, five years?

TC: Well, one of the new projects we're just in the process of creating is a mad cooperative called "Locooperativa". Basically, our idea is to help people with diagnostic labels have the opportunity to work— and with the work not framed from a "sane" perspective. So to explain: a mad perspective on work is working few hours, while having enough money to live in a decent way.

BB: So you are referring to a perspective toward work that is basically more human and more flexible?

TC: Yes, and not overworking and working at something that you like—this is a mad perspective.

BB: At the same time, a perspective that counters the forces of capitalism. That noted, what is personally on the horizon for you yourself, Tatiana?

TC: I would like to contribute more from an academic perspective. Though, you know, since being in the movement, I've substantially changed my perspective about careers.

BB: So you are not interested in being a careerist, but you are interested in creating knowledge?

TC: And you know, I don't work as an anthropologist, though this was my training. Right now I work as a receptionist.

BB: It's your day job to support your activism?

TC: Exactly. Activism is my real job.

BB: I very much get that.

TC: And the ones of us who have stayed in the movement largely share this perspective.

BB: Which means you really are bone fide activists. That said, our conversation is slowly drawing to a close. So, Tatiana, is there anything that I haven't asked you that you'd like to talk about?

TC: There's another important group that I'd like to bring up. It also came out of Libre-Mente. And it opposes the use of psychiatric drugs on children.

BB: An important development, especially with drugging of children dramatically on the rise.

TC: And it looks like this is the most winnable of our fights because folk in Chile are very uneasy about giving children psychiatric drugs. Now in the schools, of course, they push psychiatric drugs, but we have been able to mount seminars in the schools questioning this.

BB: What's the group called?

TC: It's called "For Children Being Free of Psychiatric Drugs". They meet about every two weeks and they've actually done a lot of activities in schools.

BB: So they've been invited into schools to present?

TC: Exactly.

BB: That's a highly strategic direction for schools have long served as a primary route into psychiatry.

TC: And presentations and workshops from this group have been solicited not only by teachers but also by student groups.

BB: Excellent.

TC: And the last thing that I want to mention is a project that the survivor Rodrigo is leading called "The Mad Farm". Its material basis is a property that he and his partner, I think, were given. They are intending to turn it into a place for people to go that want to get off psychiatric drugs. Where they can withdraw safely and near nature. At the same time, the Mad Farm is also a place of refuge and mutual support.

BB: That sounds really promising. And the back-to-nature dimension is important for part of our alienation is surely coming from the fact that we have pulled away from nature.

TC: Precisely.

BB: I wish Rodrigo luck with this. And on that note, Tatiana, let me thank you again for this interview. I'm pleased that a window onto the excellent Chilean initiatives is going to be part of this book.

TC: I am delighted too. Maybe it will lead to movement people from other countries starting to visit us.

BB: And it is so important that North Americans get to know what you are doing and connect with you. People in the North America movements tend to overstate their own centrality and be relatively ignorant of what is going on in the rest of the world. We know about the UK, yes, but about very little beyond that.

TC: Yeah.

BB: And if we are to have a viable movement, it needs to be truly global. And we need all of the countries represented.

TC: We need to be connected, as you say. And we don't need a revolution in what is called "mental health", but rather a larger societal revolution.

BB. Indeed, we have to live together differently. We have to respect and accommodate difference. We have to humanize, and in so doing, de professionalize. We have to find ways to resolve conflict in a communal way and to support one another. You know, many groups in the mad and the antipsychiatry movements, despite having a broad underlying philosophy, tend to limit their focus to the "mental health industry" on one hand and the celebration of madness on the other. And as such, they are not fully revolutionary. By contrast, what is happening in Chile strikes me as broader and more fundamental. Which is one of the reasons that it is critical that your initiatives and *modus operandi* become more widely known.

TC: I agree.

BB: That said, thanks again for this conversation.

REPRESENTATIVE PUBLICATIONS OF TATIANA CASTILLO

Madrid, J. C. C., & Parada, T. C. (2016). Materiales para una historia de antipsiquiatria: Balance y perspectivas. *Teoría y Crítica de la Psicología, 8,* 169–192. Downloaded August 19, 2018 from http://teocripsi.com/ojs/index.php/TCP/article/view/159/143

Parada, T. C., & Madrid, J. C. C. (2017). "Sin nosotros no hay derechos": apuntes sobre el Primer Encuentro Nacional por los Derechos Humanos de las personas en situación de discapacidad mental en Chile. *Revista Latinoamericana en Discapacidad, Sociedad y Derechos Humanos, 1*(1). Downloaded August 19, 2018 from http://redcdpd.net/revista/index.php/revista/article/view/34

TATIANA'S ADDED COMMENT

A few clarifying words about several of the more prominent movement groups in Chile: The collective *Autogestión Libre-Mente* represents a participatory community space in "mental health". It holds open meetings every Monday in an anarchist social center located in the downtown area of Santiago. The primary folk participating are those who have lived an experience of having a diagnosis and "psychiatric treatment", along with people who consider themselves allies. Attendance is free and each meeting is facilitated by a mental health user or ex-user/survivor. The aim is to develop and integrate alternatives to "psychiatry", to promote the recognition of people's rights in "mental health", and to use the potential of community spaces to foster a sense of collective well-being. In practice, the values of horizontality, reciprocity, and solidarity as axes of shared dialogue allow the collective to function as a mutual support group.

"Mad for Our Rights" is a collective formed by experts by experience (users and ex-users of "mental health" services) and experts by formation (professionals in the social sciences area). They created a publication called "Manual of Rights in Mental Health", which integrates a global view about the importance of rights in the mental health field from the perspective of the community of users and ex-users. They have made more than 80 presentations related to the *Manual of Rights in Mental Health* in community spaces, "mental health" institutions, and universities throughout Chile. Since its publication in 2015, the manual has become an enormously useful instrument of social transformation, since it is the only document published in Chile from an expert by experience perspective [anyone wanting a copy of this manual is urged to write to: locospornuestrosderechoes@gmail.com].

"Free Lectures Franco Basaglia" [*Cátedra Libre Franco Basaglia*] is an academic discussion space oriented toward the social and political aspects of the "mental health" field. The Cátedra has created activities to raise awareness that electroshock is a damaging and harmful practice, and it has as well created forums which problematize the use of psychiatric drugs.

The Mad Studies Center is a platform which brings mad and "sane" people together to develop investigative projects within university settings and to build knowledge in the defense of the right to madness. The success of this initiative is manifested in its ability to draw together professionals, mad folks, and students on both a national and international level.

Follow the collectives on Facebook:

Autogestión Libre-Mente
Locos por nuestros derechos
Centro de estudios locos
Cátedra Libre Franco Basaglia
No es lo mismo ser loca que loco

Por una niñez libre de drogas psiquiátricas

CHAPTER 9

"There Is No Place on This Planet for Psychiatry Period!": Dialogue with Don Weitz

An activist since the 1970s, Don Weitz is the heart and soul of antipsychiatry. He co-founded the first antipsychiatry magazine in North America— Phoenix Rising. *He likewise co-founded many antipsychiatry organizations. Moreover, he is a prolific author, and indeed co-editor along with me, of the historic* Shrink Resistant *(Burstow and Weitz 1988)—the world's first anthology of survivor stories. A firm believer in demonstrations, even now in his late 80s, Don can frequently be found protesting, megaphone in hand.*

Don and my connection is extensive. Friends and allies, we have co-written, co-edited, and co-organized since the very early 1980s. Both of us disabled now, when we came to do this interview, the conflict between our disabilities was quickly apparent. As someone partially deaf, Don needed me to repeat almost everything I said; correspondingly, as someone with a pronounced sensitivity to sound, I kept asking him to talk softer. However, we both soldiered on, leading to the exchange below:

BB: Of all my interviewees, you're by far the one I know the best. We've been antipsychiatry comrades working side by side for decades. Let's eventually revisit some of the places we've been together. But I wanted to start with something very specific to you—how Don Weitz—the antipsychiatry activist that we all know and love—came to be who he is. Maybe it would help if I made an

© The Author(s) 2019

B. Burstow, *The Revolt Against Psychiatry*,
https://doi.org/10.1007/978-3-030-23331-0_9

121

observation: A large number of people become antipsychiatry activists having been survivors—and that is certainly part of your history. However, there is another part of your history that is truly extraordinary. That is, you became an antipsychiatry activist having first been a psychologist. So how is it that Don Weitz psychologist became Don Weitz—psychiatric survivor activist?

DW: (laughing): You know what happened? I was so brain-washed that I wanted to become a professional and I went to university to do this. At that time I believed in the medical model. Like many others, I believed there was such a thing as mental illness. So I pursued a masters in psychology. Then I got a job in Cleveland Psychiatric Institute, testing people labeled schizophrenic.

BB: Testing them for what?

DW: To see if they were crazy. Well (laughing), what I was administering were psychological tests. And I took pride in acting very professionally. This was 1956–57. And in 62 I moved from the States to Canada, where I became a psychology instructor at Centennial College [Toronto community college], still believing in what I was doing. In 1970, I joined Queen St. Mental Health Centre [a huge provincial mental health center in downtown Toronto] as a community psychologist. Now I worked at an outpatient clinic but I also worked on the wards as a so-called counselor.

BB: In the belly of the beast? 999 Queen West?

DW: 999 Queen. What I witnessed there is that many of the patients labeled uncontrollable were being put into a physical restraint device called "the cold wet pack". Bonnie, it was horrible to witness. Literally, they were wrapped up in their beds like mummies in cold wet sheets and kept there for hours, sometimes days.

BB: So you were horrified by it?

DW: And angry as hell that staff would use and condone this physical restraining device when it was blatantly torturous. So I wrote a letter to the head of the therapeutic standards committee, requesting it be stopped.

BB: What was the response?

DW: He sent me back a very short note—"thank you for your concern"— a typical bureaucratic response. Of course, it didn't stop anything. So I asked the psychology department where I worked to speak up about it. The chief psychologist refused. The other psychologists refused. Whereupon, I became more outraged.

BB: And it got you questioning psychology too, I take it, for you were seeing that psychology was in bed with psychiatry, had been coopted by psychiatry?

DW: Yes. Psychiatrists and psychologists were partners.

BB: So is this when you started to have doubts about being a psychologist?

DW: More than doubts. I was experiencing moral agony. I would wake up in the middle of the night asking myself: How can I work at a place like this? How can I be part of such a profession? And I quit in September 1972.

BB: Very few people, never mind professionals, face up to the reality of what they are a part of, and I so respect that. That said, of those that do, even less quit—for the investment is huge—and fewer still become activists. Don, how did that come about?

DW: I asked myself: What the hell kind of system is this that tortures people? I also knew that forced drugging and electroshock was going on at the time and that it too was torturous. So I started to read Thomas Szasz (1961). His book [*The Myth of Mental Illness*], you know, came out in 1961 and I said: Exactly. I also read Leonard Frank [electroshock survivor who was an authoritative critic of electroshock]. The first psychiatric survivor magazine *Madness Network News* [see http://www.madnessnetworknews.com/], was going strong, and I read what Frank wrote there—and that gave me courage to speak out.

BB: And soon, you were not speaking out as a professional but rather speaking out as a survivor? How did that transition happen?

DW: Not sure what you're asking.

BB: How did you stop identifying as a professional and begin identifying as a psychiatric survivor?

DW: I took a trip out to the Mental Patients Association in B.C., which was Canada's first empowering survivor-controlled group. They were trying out alternatives, and I thought there had to be an alternative to the cold wet pack, forced drugging, and ECT.

BB: Given this was a place of refuge for survivors, I take it that you went not only to explore other options—a good thing in itself—but also because you were starting to look with new eyes at your early life, perhaps beginning to reclaim identity in a new way?

DW: I started to have an internal conversation with myself.

BB: And in the process you stopped identifying as a professional?

124   B. BURSTOW

DW: Yes. You see, in my youth, I had been locked up and "treated" 110 times with insulin shock.

BB: Horrible. I'm so sorry.

DW: When I was just going through a normal adolescent identity crisis. Now at the time I was traumatized, but as time passed, I started to identify with the oppressor.

BB: By which you mean the psychiatrists?

DW: Yes.

BB: And identifying with the oppressor, you became a psychologist. Then you witnessed what you could not live with, whereupon you bit by bit re-evaluated everything and took back the identity of a survivor—and now one committed to social justice. Am I putting this together correctly?

DW: Yes, I started to get in touch with my oppressed self. It took me 20 years, Bonnie. I was so traumatized. After getting out of Maclean's in 1953 [a U.S. psychiatric "hospital"], for the next 5 years I saw nine different psychiatrists, then went on to become a psychologist. But after I witnessed the cold wet pack at 999, I started to look back at my life and I said to myself: Look what's happened to you. And look at what's happening to so many others. Why are you being quiet? Why aren't you being active? So that's how it is that I started to identify with my oppression. Then I took that trip out west and got in touch with politicized survivors. They were so supportive. I stayed a week at the MPA House [Mental Patient's Association House, a supportive place where survivors could stay], which was run totally democratically. Then I returned to Toronto and asked myself: Why can't we create something like that here?

BB: Which I take it is how the survivor support group On Our Own [the first psychiatric survivor support group in Ontario] came into being?

DW: On Our Own was formed in 1977 at the instigation of Bob Carson, Alf Jackson, and me [all Toronto psychiatric survivors]. We started a group for survivors like ourselves, with the idea of helping people stay out of the system.

BB: An amazing transition, Don, though my sense is that this survivor protest identity was in you all along. You know, when I was writing *Psychiatry and the Business of Madness* [Burstow 2015], you were one of the two people who gave me your hospital records.

9 "THERE IS NO PLACE ON THIS PLANET FOR PSYCHIATRY PERIOD!"... 125

DW: That's right.

BB: Now right in the hospital transcript itself, I could see traces of the important survivor activist that you would later become. This being a psychiatric record, of course, what I encountered were very judgmental remarks by staff. Nonetheless, in the very behavior that they pathologized was a story that begged to be read differently. They used the word "obsessive" to describe the fact that you always examined ideas from multiple angles—whereas I thought to myself—don't they realize that this is what intellectuals do? And they took your anger at being subjected to insulin shock as psychosis instead of what it was—the beginnings of a moral revolt.

DW: Exactly.

BB: That said, what really got to me when I read the transcript was that this youth was being subjected to insulin shock over and over [an early convulsive "treatment"]. What was it like for you? And how do you think that this experience influenced you later as an activist?

DW: It certainly educated me about the use of coercion. Also it allowed me to see that this is a profession that really hurts people. What was it like? I was in agony.

BB: Yes, I could see that. And according to the records, a number of times the staff didn't even know whether or not they were going to be able to bring you back from the near-death state in which they had placed you. And yet they relentlessly persisted.

DW: And I was vocally protesting. And I was in physical and emotional pain for 6 consecutive weeks.

BB: So sorry, Don. Can I check out a hunch here? Your biggest single focus as an activist appears to be the struggle to end "electroconvulsive therapy". And I've always thought that one of things that attracted you so strongly to this focus—not that you need another reason to oppose something so obviously unacceptable—is that you yourself had experienced insulin shock.

DW: That's right. I could see the similarities. It was also about doing something brutal to the person.

BB: Yes, and as you were well aware, it too was a treatment predicated on forcing a convulsion on the person. In fact, electroshock was the very next of the convulsive treatments, the next rendition of "convulsive therapy". So my guess is that you must have felt and perhaps still do feel a special kinship to ECT [electroshock] survivors.

DW: Oh yeah. I could see the similarities clearly.

BB: Which brings us to your anti-ECT activism. You and I have worked side by side for decades in a number of different groups committed to stopping ECT—Ontario Coalition to Stop Electroshock etc. What do you see as our most effective actions? And what were our most serious mistakes?

DW: Well, in August of 1983 as Ontario Coalition to Stop Electroshock, one memorable thing we did is organize hearings against electroshock at Toronto City Hall, where shock survivors got to testify—and it is always empowering for people to speak out. And that led to a demonstration against the Clark Institute of Psychiatry [known as the "shock shop" of Ontario]. You know, we were brilliant activists, were terrific at educating the general public and our brothers and sisters.

BB: So we were good at helping people speak out and good at consciousness-raising?

DW: And we held a number of effective public protests. Very effective—and it really garnered the attention of the press. Take the act of civil disobedience in which you, Shirley Johnson [electroshock survivor], and me did a sit-in in the Minister of Health's office.

BB: Yes, historically, the very first sit-in of any kind in an Ontario minister's office. And for sure we garnered considerable coverage.

DW: (beaming) A historical and a thrilling moment.

BB: For sure. At the same time, let's flip this over. We didn't actually succeed in changing what happens to people at the hands of shock doctors. So yes, while we have much to be proud of, in retrospect, is there anything that you think we might have done better?

DW: Perhaps if we had networked more so as to get more clout politically. We were probably too insular.

BB: And is your sense in general that one of the places antipsychiatry errs is insufficiently networking with other social justice groups?

DW: Yes, though this is a shortcoming common to most social movement groups, and we nonetheless made important breakthroughs. We helped folk tell their story publicly.

BB: We did indeed. And I've never seen anything since even vaguely close to the quality of public testimony that we got. People like Shirley Johnson and Connie Neil [leading Ontario shock survivors] were overwhelmingly powerful.

9 "THERE IS NO PLACE ON THIS PLANET FOR PSYCHIATRY PERIOD!"... 127

DW: And remember the quality of the statements that we made before the Toronto Board of Health months earlier. You spoke out as a professional. And Ralph Preston spoke [survivor and physicist].

BB: Yes, and we did well. That said, let me tell you the biggest mistake that I think we made—for I'm convinced it's as important to learn from our mistakes as to celebrate our victories—we called for an investigation into ECT. That's different than demanding it be stopped. All they had to do was form a committee to investigate shock and the story that we'd worked so hard at orchestrating would be dead. Which is exactly what they did. So they said, fine, we'll give you an investigation. So for two years they investigated, and long before the investigation came to an end, the ECT story was "yesterday's news". So while on one level, I agree we did amazing work—we helped survivors speak out and we got the attention of the public—on another, the truth is that we really weren't savvy activists. One of the ABC's of grass roots activism is never to ask for an investigation but always and only to demand change. One of my great regrets is, we didn't know that.

DW: Yes, we should instead have upped the ante with direct action.

BB: So when you say we were brilliant activists, let me suggest that at the time, we weren't.

DW: Well, we did make demands when we were Resistance Against Psychiatry [next antipsychiatry group in Ontario].

BB: True, but by that time, we had already lost the press.

DW: You know, Bonnie, we could have learned from the Berkeley group [a US group that got shock stopped for 40 days via a referendum—until the courts overturned the decision]. They were more active than us. Not that they were antipsychiatry. We were the only ones in Ontario who were psychiatry abolitionists.

BB: Actually, at the time we were the only group *anywhere* that was fully abolitionist. Let's be clear. When it comes to vision, we were light years ahead of everyone else. And we owe a large part of that to you.

DW: It did not take me long to think and act antipsychiatry. And then there was you. You were the only "academic" and the only professional who not only denounced psychiatry but called for abolition. And we did that in print as well through *Phoenix Rising*.

BB: When I look at it, we Toronto antipsychiatry folks kept antipsychiatry alive at a time when almost no one else was taking this position. We essentially held the space that needed to be held. Something that made the current swell in antipsychiatry possible.

DW: Yes, we had the courage of our convictions. Others were scared to go that far. And I would say: Why the hell not? If an oppressor is stepping on your neck, you don't take half measures. Now to go back to shock, I think we have to reframe the struggle against shock as primarily a human rights struggle.

BB: Which reminds me, one of the other strengths you have brought to this struggle is that you were one of the people who consistently stressed psychiatry's systemic violation of human rights. Like David Oaks, like Leonard Roy Frank [legendary American survivor activists].

DW: Absolutely.

BB: A position which was front and center in the various international conferences bearing the name "International Conference on Human Rights and Psychiatric Oppression". It comes across particularly strongly in the 1982 principles passed at the Tenth Annual Conference on Human Rights and Psychiatric Oppression [see https://www.madinamerica.com/forums/topic/statement-of-principles-from-10th-annual-conference-on-human-rights/]

DW: Something again held in Toronto.

BB: And what most people fail to recognize is that interfering with people's choices, locking them up, plying them with drugs that they do not want in itself constitutes a basic human right violation, as the United Nations has made abundantly clear [see Convention on the Rights of Persons with Disabilities at https://www.un.org/development/desa/disabilities/convention-on-the-rights-of-persons-with-disabilities.html]

DW: Yes, and this can't be stressed enough.

BB: To focus back in once again on shock, let me ask you something: Do you think that there is a special role that the protest against ECT plays or can play either for the survivor movement or for the antipsychiatry movement?

DW: Definitely. Why? Because the harm and the violation is so blatant.

BB: So blatant that it functions as a symbol of what is wrong with psychiatry overall, much like the reality of the cold wet pack functioned for you all those years ago. And my own take is that given

9 "THERE IS NO PLACE ON THIS PLANET FOR PSYCHIATRY PERIOD!"... 129

the symbolism, the struggle against ECT is a very apt one to lead with.

DW: Yes. ECT is grounded in violence—and in it you see the paradigm, as you often put it. Future organizing, I would suggest, should be stressing the institutionalization of violence.

BB: Nicely put, Don. To move on, when I look at your primary focus currently, I am aware that in many ways you've come full circle. You left the profession of psychology in least partially because of restraints—cold wet packs etc. And these days, you are focusing in on the use of seclusion—a similar phenomenon.

DW: I'm glad you brought that up, Bonnie, for that also is violence. Seclusion is violence being perpetrated by two interrelated systems—the psychiatric system and the prison system. But at least when it comes to the prison system, investigative reporters expose it. Not so with the psychiatric system.

BB: Yes, and we both know, the problem is not just psychiatry but psychology, and not just these two professions but the industries that feed them and which they in turn support—moreover—and this speaks to the lack of real investigative reporting—the media itself is inherently complicit.

DW: So we have to demonstrate against all of it.

BB: Agreed, but that's not enough. Demonstrations alone will not change the system. As we know from the paucity of coverage since the 1990s, nor does it necessarily even garner the press. Now to be clear I don't think demonstrations are even close to the total answer, but let's pretend for a moment that they are. How do we fashion demonstrations so that the media turns up?

DW: That's a challenge in organizing. We have to brainstorm new approaches to organizing. And we have to return to direct action. We have to challenge the very legitimacy of the psychiatric system.

BB: Ah, but we have.

DW: We have in books, but when it comes to organizing, I don't think the organizing in the US or Canada has ever made the systemic visible. We need an attack on the system itself.

BB: Say more. How does one demonstrate against the whole system?

DW: Maybe if we had an international approach.

BB: Okay, let's look at that. We had a huge international protest against shock a couple of years ago [the 2015 International Day of Protest against Electroshock Treatment—see https://www.facebook.com/events/880990481961272/]. And did the press cover it? Barely!

130   B. BURSTOW

DW: The point is, though, there needs to be an international protest not simply against shock but against all of psychiatry. In Germany, there have been effective protests where the very premise, very ideology of psychiatry has been challenged. Now if we could get people together to organize in this fundamental way in France, in Germany, in Canada, in the US, in Argentina, in Brazil, that could be the route, but to do it well, we'd have first have an international conference. Now I know we've had international conferences. Actually in Toronto, we were one of the first.

BB: Yes, PsychOut [the very first international conference focused specifically on activism; see https://coalitionagainstpsychiatricassault.wordpress.com/events/past-events/psychout-a-conference-for-organizing-resistance-against-psychiatry/].

DW: Yes and it was a start, Bonnie. But it has to be expanded. We need a mega international conference where we get activists from across the world to stand together, and we need to take on every aspect of the system.

BB: I see your vision, Don, and naturally, I respect it. At the same time, I'm aware that to realize it, we would have to have far greater numbers.

DW: We need *hundreds* involved.

BB: We *did have hundreds* at the PsychOut Conference.

DW: Correction, we need *thousands*.

BB: But how do we get the thousands, and how do we organize so that thousands keep up the pressure, surely that's the question. Exactly how do we pull that off?

DW: Well, part of what we need to do is highlight alternatives. Now we already have exciting pilot experiments and sustainable alternatives in several countries. And we have to showcase these and let the world know that survivors and their allies themselves have created these successful nonmedical alternatives.

BB: For the sake of readers unfamiliar with these, Don, could you give an example?

DW: Well, there's Runaway House—it's a place [see Chap. 6] where people can go where there is no schedule and whose main purpose is to help people stay out of the psychiatric system. It serves a mix of people—people who have been in the system and don't want to end up back there, people who have snuck out when no one's looking, those who have never been in but have been threatened

9 "THERE IS NO PLACE ON THIS PLANET FOR PSYCHIATRY PERIOD!"... 131

by the system. It still exists. And there are little or no drugs used. Self-help is pivotal, as are the dissident professionals involved. The big thing is, it is very informal, and there is no coercion whatever. It was similar really to what got created in the US. What was its name?

BB: Soteria House [a relatively drug-free American option for people labeled "schizophrenic" started by leading US "schizophrenia" expert Loren Mosher in 1971; see https://en.wikipedia.org/wiki/Soteria_] So that's part of what you would like to see? More energy put into options with a proven track record? And here we hit into yet another snag that we need to come to terms with as activists. The point is, one of the things we know about the original Soteria House is that it worked so incredibly well that the authorities closed it down, for it was clear proof of a reality that the establishment did not want known: that so-called schizophrenics do not need to be on drugs—indeed, do better if they aren't. And herein lies the difficulty: In North America anyway—fortunately not at the moment in Berlin—cutting off funding, that's what the authorities do when something non-medical is shown to really work—an easy thing to do in this particular case, for Mosher's funding came from National Institute of Mental Health [the US governmental body whose job it is to further research in line with the medical model; see https://www.nimh.nih.gov/about/index.shtml].

DW: Yes, and so as you yourself have often said, we need to have independent community funding. Funding and accountability outside the "mental health" system.

BB: Absolutely. Which is part of the genius at work when they founded Berlin Runaway House, for they secured funding from a completely different part of government. So are you suggesting that those of us who oppose psychiatry should be looking at creating our own home-grown services? Perhaps not funded by the government at all?

DW: Yes.

BB: You are essentially thinking of services at a grass roots community level?

DW: Precisely.

132   B. BURSTOW

BB: I couldn't agree more. Don, thank you for sharing your wisdom today. Before we close, is there anything further you want to discuss?

DW: Just to reemphasize the importance of planning a mega-conference. More generally, we need people from all walks of life, including dissident psychiatrists, to join together in huge numbers and say that there is no place on this planet for the profession of psychiatry—*period*!

BB: Old friend and comrade, much thanks.

REFERENCES

Burstow, B. (2015). *Psychiatry and the business of madness.* New York: Palgrave Macmillan.

Burstow, B., & Weitz, D. (Eds.). (1988). *Shrink resistant: The struggle against psychiatry in Canada.* Vancouver: New Star Press.

Szasz, T. (1961). *The myth of mental illness.* New York: Paul B. Hoeber.

REPRESENTATIVE PUBLICATIONS BY DON WEITZ

Burstow, B., & Weitz, D. (Eds.). (1988). *Shrink resistant: The struggle against psychiatry in Canada.* Vancouver: New Star Books.

Weitz, D. (1997). Electroshocking elderly people: Another psychiatric abuse. *Changes: An International Journal of Psychology and Psychotherapy, 15*(2), 118–123.

Weitz, D. (1998, February). Here's to Alf. *Canadian Dimension.*

Weitz, D. (2003). Call me "antipsychiatry activist"—Not "consumer". *Ethical Human Sciences and Services, 5*(1), 71–72.

Weitz, D. (2004). Insulin shock: A survivor's account of psychiatric torture. *Journal of Critical Psychology, Counselling, and Psychotherapy, 4*(3).

Weitz, D. (2008a). *End electroshock now—An antipsychiatry perspective.* www.psychiatrized.org/DonWeitz/End%20ElectroshockNow.pdf

Weitz, D. (2008b). Struggling against psychiatry's human rights violations: An antipsychiatry perspective. *Radical/Psychology, 7.*

Weitz, D. (2010). *Electroshock must be banned now: Strategies of resistance.* A paper presented at PsychOut: A Conference for Organizing Resistance Against Psychiatry. www.individual.utoronto.ca/psychout/panels/weitz_paper.pdf

Weitz, D. (2011). *Rise up/fight back: Selected writings of an antipsychiatry activist.* E-book.   www.amazon.ca/Rise-Up-Fight-Back-Antipsychiatry-ebook/dp/B007EIBK0K

Weitz, D. (2013). Electroshock: Torture as treatment. In B. LeFrançois, R. Menzies, & G. Reaume (Eds.), *Mad matters: A critical reader in Canadian mad studies* (pp. 258–169). Toronto: Canadian Scholars Press.

Weitz, D., Crowe, C., Moodley, R., Dunphy, C., & Rahim, C. (2005). *Electroshock is not a healing option: Report of the panel, enquiry into psychiatry.* www.coalitionagainstpsychiatricassault.files.wordpress.com/2010/09/shockreport.pdf

Weitz, D., Maddock, M., & Andre, L. (2010). *Strategies to ban electroshock.* A paper presented at PsychOut: A Conference for Organizing Resistance Against Psychiatry. www.individual.utoronto.ca/psychout/abstracts/weitz-etal.html

CHAPTER 10

Autistic and Mad: Dialogue with Nick Walker

Nick Walker is an autistic university teacher and a major theorist in the neurodiversity movement. Nick is also the co-founder and managing editor of a radical publishing house called Autonomous Press (see http://autpress. com/). Correspondingly, his shorter writings on neurodiversity and cognitive liberty can be found on his blog Neurocosmopolitanism (see http://neurocos-mopolitanism.com).

The two of us are united by a common goal to bring the mad/antipsychiatry movement and the neurodiversity movement closer together. Last time Nick and I were in a project together, we were the guest podcasters on a Mad in America *podcast called "Bonnie Burstow and Nick Walker: An Introduction to Cognitive Liberty" (see https://www.madinamerica.com/2017/10/ bonnie-burstow-nick-walker/).*

BB: Welcome to this project, Nick. Nice to be talking to you again. You are a leader in the neurodiversity movement, correct?

NW: Not exactly. I don't identify as a leader or an activist. What I am is a major theorist, building the theory necessary.

BB: Understood. Now I know you identify as mad, autistic, and queer. Also starting in childhood, you've had a huge number of psychiatric labels.

NW: I wasn't actually diagnosed as autistic until adulthood. And much later, when autistic got brought up, I recognized myself in the

© The Author(s) 2019
B. Burstow, *The Revolt Against Psychiatry*,
https://doi.org/10.1007/978-3-030-23331-0_10

135

description. As a child, it was psychiatric diagnoses that I received. I was one of first people to be diagnosed with Oppositional Defiant Disorder, this when I was 12.

BB: A horrible and judgmental diagnosis but if looked at from outside how the system wants you to look at it, in some ways a very reassuring diagnosis, for what it means is that you were not accepting the crap that adults were putting on you.

NW: Absolutely.

BB: You know what amazes and thrills me here? As a brilliant young boy, a) you saw that there was something wrong with these diagnoses; and b) you realized it was actually better not to fit into the expectations placed on you. How soon did you begin to figure this out?

NW: From age 9 onward, I was acutely aware that it was not me but the dominant, allegedly sane culture that was broken and rigid and full of hate and fear. And those of us that were "crazy", mad, and queer, and divergent, we were free of that. And indeed, we were a threat to the established order.

BB: And you realized that how you thought and acted was preferable to fitting into the established order?

NW: Absolutely preferable.

BB: That you started to realize this at 9 years old is incredible, also reassuring. Because the message that society drums into the heads of children is that if they are not marching in step, the problem is them. That said, I am curious here. How did you parents react? Did they reject what the establishment was putting on you?

NW: How to explain this? My parents were negligent.

BB: Did they subject you to the terrible operant conditioning that happens to children?

NW: They didn't. That's the lovely part of their negligence.

BB: So the benefit of their negligence is that you escaped the treatment (read "abuse") inflicted on children given such diagnoses?

NW: Exactly. My parents were very young when I was born and not well equipped to parent. Negligent, with abuse coming from my father's trauma rather than systemic abuse. There was no attempt to make me normal.

BB: So while horrible things befell you in childhood, you escaped the normalization regime systematically inflicted on "mentally ill" and autistic children?

NW: Yes, though again, I wasn't recognized as autistic at the time. You know, at the time, it was uncommon for kids to be diagnosed as autistic unless they were non-speaking, whereas I was highly articulate some of the time, while at other times I did not speak. And because I was highly articulate, no one noticed when I couldn't speak.

BB: I see. But you weren't spared the other diagnoses given to children. And they diagnosed you with Oppositional Defiant Disorder.

NW: Also with various other "personality disorders".

BB: And you somehow knew that what was being invalidated in this way were very good parts of yourself?

NW: Precisely. I knew that the society which doles out these diagnoses is not to be trusted. Anyway, as I grew older, I ended up discovering artists who were considered crazy and were defiant, also authors like George Orwell who wrote eloquently about how oppression is structured. And those discoveries have always been a tremendous asset to me. You know, most other people who are mad, queer, or neurodivergent struggle with internalized oppression. Even people transparently into Autistic Pride and Mad Pride tend to be plagued by terrible anxiety and self-doubt. As in: Am I really okay? Did I just do something wrong? And that does not happen to me—because I worked through all of that in early childhood.

BB: An amazing feat that surely set you up to be the important theorist that you are. Now as you developed as a theorist, you quickly took up the term "neurodiversity". What it is about that word that spoke to you?

NW: Well, when I was in my early 30s, I finally got diagnosed as autistic. And I realized, yes, that is the core piece that I was missing. And you know, I was working as a reading tutor with autistic kids at the time and what happened is I recognized the similarity in how we lived in the world. So I sought out the diagnosis myself.

BB: What is it about the actual word that you liked?

NW: Well, I was already thinking of autism and so forth as a diversity issue. Anyway, the word "neurodiversity" was coined in 1998, and I stumbled upon it in 2002, and I thought to myself: Yes, this word sums everything up. What we have here is a type of diversity that involves the same dynamics as other forms of human diversity, including power relations and dominant groups oppressing minorities.

138   B. BURSTOW

BB: Absolutely, and it took you into a world where "we are all different"—and into the position that "difference is good".

NW: Yes, so I became an early adopter of the word. And I quickly began spreading the word and clarifying the definitions and implications of the word. Hence my evolution as a neurodiversity theorist.

BB: Now in your writing and speaking, you emphasize such issues as the importance of scrapping the medical paradigm.

NW: Exactly. I contrast the pathology paradigm, which is all about disease, and the neurodiversity paradigm, which is about natural difference.

BB: To shift topics slightly, every social movement is plagued with incredible tensions. And I wonder how you strategize in relation to this. Take a recent blog critique pronouncing the neurodiversity movement dead [this blog article is not being referenced so as not to give it publicity]. What is your strategy for dealing with attacks like this? Like, did you ask yourself: How can I respond to blog articles like this in a way that has the potential of bringing naysayers on side?

NW: Actually, when I see ridiculous arguments leveled against the neurodiversity paradigm or Mad Pride activism, or queer activism, I just remind myself that there is nothing new here, and since I'm not an activist, I need not respond. I have put the ideas out there. I have published them online in easily digestible articles. And any activist who wants to quote them or post links to them can do so.

BB: So you're saying you don't engage with critics?

NW: I would if I ever encountered a critic who had an original argument. And I have yet to encounter that. Now I know I am making a controversial statement here because so much of activist culture is about jumping into the fray, especially these days where so much happens on social media. There is always an on-line war going on somewhere. I am unconcerned. And let me suggest in this day and age where everyone is charged up and ready to jump in on conflicts at the drop of a hat, it is a radical act to be unconcerned. As I see it, I'm helping to engineer a social paradigm shift—from the pathology paradigm to the neurodiversity paradigm—and all that is associated with it, which for me includes mad pride and concepts like cognitive liberty.

BB: You are drawing on Thomas Kuhn [1962] when you use the word "paradigm", aren't you?

NW:	Yes. And Kuhn had something extremely valuable to say about paradigm shifts. Namely, that very few people make a paradigm shift in their lifetime. What happens is that the ideas are out there and eventually, the people attached to the old paradigm die off.
BB:	He likewise points out that the work of scientists is to resolve anomalies in prevailing paradigms, which becomes less attractive as awareness of the anomalies grow. And, of course, raising that awareness is certainly what has been going on within the antipsychiatry, mad, and neurodiversity communities.
NW:	Exactly. And that's what we are seeing now. We have a culture which is rampant with unresolved anomalies. Where all the old norms have collapsed.
BB:	To a significant degree, yes, but the power structures are still there, and people still pay attention to those old norms. Look at the power of psychiatry and psychology to this day.
NW:	How I see it is: Lots of people are desperately clinging to old paradigms and trying to enforce them but there is an aggressiveness in how they cling to them that tells me they are embattled.
BB:	An insightful and very apt point, that.
NW:	In this post-normal era, everyone is fighting tooth-and-nail for some degree of certainty and it's not sustainable. People are frantic because their illusions of certainty are threatened. And I see that in psychiatry as well. And all the while, these institutional players become caricatures of themselves.
BB:	Yes, and especially in these days of the so-called scientific DSM, which has been proven to be unscientific repeatedly.
NW:	So when I see these skirmishes, and I see people bring up these same invalid arguments over and over, I think: I don't have to respond. I just have to wait for them to die.
BB:	(laughing) Spoken like a long-term visionary. You trust in the future being with you and not with them.
NW:	You see, I've practiced aikido for a long time, and the principles of aikido inform my approach in that I don't feel the need to respond to anything that I don't see as a serious threat.
BB:	So what I see you as doing is laying the foundations for the collapse of the paradigm, then patiently waiting for the system to collapse. Now correct me if I'm mistaken, but isn't it hard sticking only with that long-term way of operating when you are seeing more and more people getting hurt? So, for instance, do you not

140 B. BURSTOW

ever end up thinking that what with the rapid growth of the use of electroshock on autistic children in Great Britain, a more immediate response is also in order?

NW: Absolutely, but not by me. So I put my analyses on line so that they can be understood and cited. And that's what I see as my part of the job. By contrast, it is the job of people who see themselves as activists to weigh in in the here-and-now. That said, you know, there's a limit to what activists can actually do. What is happening to children is terrible, but we cannot literally save each one. We don't have an army that can stop the torturers.

BB: True, but we can draw attention to and object to what is happening. What if we devoted some energy to pushing the UN, for instance, to declare the electroshocking of children a human rights violation?

NW: Sure, there is a place for an activist response, though the major thing for me is that's not my niche. My work involves creating the theoretic foundations, though also I'm now involved in practices to heal the community. One thing that is clear about the autistic movement and the mad movement, we are deeply traumatized communities. And because so many of the individual activists are deeply traumatized, they are easily triggered. And we have people acting out their traumas. As a result, the activist community itself can be horrifically abusive. People attack each other.

BB: So what sort of things have you been doing to counter that? Or, as you put it, to "heal the community"?

NW: You know, I am in an interesting place for I am autistic, mad, and queer, but I'm also a psychologist and a college professor who trains future psychotherapists.

BB: We overlap here, for I am a university professor who trains graduate students how to work in helpful and counter-hegemonic ways with trauma survivors.

NW: Now I'm a pariah in much of the autistic activist community because I object to the ways they attack everyone and I often decline to work with them, including when it comes to writing. You know, I am co-founder and managing editor of Autonomous Press. We're a worker-owned collective, and we publish in the areas of neurodivergence, madness, and queerness. Now we initially wanted to publish works of lots of autistic activists, but we find many of them too hostile. Bottom line, we won't work with people who have a history of attacking others on social media.

BB: I get that. Now one of the strengths of your press is you made a commitment to make visible more autistic voices. So autistic people making and speaking their own theory, instead of being theorized by others.

NW: Yes, and not just autistic but queer, mad, and neurodivergent people of all sorts.

BB: You know what, Nick? Personally, I see this publishing initiative as a form of activism—you are helping give voice to people who are not supposed to have a voice.

NW: (laughter) Understood, and I'll admit to being that type of activist.

BB: (laughter) To go back to the issue of movements, you are bringing together the mad movement and the autistic movement, and given your personal story, it is a natural thing for you to do for you know in a personal way the oppression of both.

NW: And I don't draw a hard line between these phenomena.

BB: Nor should there be hard lines. Nonetheless, for many people in the respective movements, there are. And so I was wondering: How do you think that these movements can be brought closer together? To give you some of the context behind this question, I have noticed that when there are blogs about autism in *Mad in America*, commenters from the mad and the antipsychiatry community often rhyme in saying something like: This is a very different issue for there is actually something physical going on with autism; so it's qualitatively different than "mental illness", which is bogus and has no physical correlate. How do you see dealing with that response? As I see it, the problem here is not only that they aren't understanding theorists like you, they're not understanding how an oppression can be configured differently.

NW: They also have no understanding of basic neuroscience. Anything that is madness is a manifestation of neurodiversity because that's how brains operate, right? If you're mad, you are thinking differently from members of the dominant culture.

BB: You are, but most of the people in the antipsychiatry movement would say: Yes, mad people are thinking differently, but there is nothing physical involved here.

NW: But they're just plain wrong. It is clear from neuroscience 101 that all of our thoughts manifest as neural pathways. If you are thinking differently …

BB: In the very process of doing this, you are altering your neurology?

NW: Exactly. It is not possible to think outside the norm without building neural pathways in your brain.

BB: Agreed.

NW: And once again, I don't see any need to engage with people who are completely wrong. It's like engaging with flat-earthers. You can't make the earth flat no matter how many people you bring to believe it is flat. And every mad brain is a neurodivergent brain, which is different from someone's whose thoughts stay within cultural norms.

BB: Understood, and at the same time, what your answer ignores is that the antipsychiatry movement has made huge strides by demonstrating that if you examine the brains of, say, people called schizophrenic, you will find that they do not differ chemically from the brains of people not so labeled. And so all the claims about chemical imbalances, and other such alleged physical "causes" are incorrect.

NW: Oh, I certainly don't believe the chemical imbalances crap.

BB: But that is exactly why people in the antipsychiatry movement tend to feel threatened by your analysis. Because antipsychiatry rests on the claim of all these so-called physical differences being bogus. At which point, it is hard for them to entertain very different types of physical claims, even when these claims have nothing to do with physical causation. Do you see what I'm saying? That does not make them flat-earthers. It makes them people defending against a particular type of position. What I am saying here, is that you can understand why people in the antipsychiatry movement would be wary of this physical way of conceptualizing things, given the history of what they have quite rightly been objecting to.

NW: Interesting. I do understand, and in that way, "neurodiversity" is actually an imperfect term for it leads to essentialization as if these were absolute brain differences rather than as an embodied way of being-in-the-world. It simply gets essentialized as neurobiology, and I push back against that too. And I get the enormity of the problem with that. You know, I think that the concept of mental illness and the concept of chemical imbalances in the brain is predicated on the false assumption that there is a correct balance in the brain.

10 AUTISTIC AND MAD: DIALOGUE WITH NICK WALKER 143

BB: I understand, and we are agreed here. At the same time, I am inviting you to appreciate the different priorities of antipsychiatry folk, who are involved in a somewhat different battle than yours.

NW: I'm not in a fight. I'm building something.

BB: Fair enough. Let me put what I was trying to say this way: The movements in question are faced with different contexts. And if we want to bring the movements together, we have to respect those differences. Which is markedly different than dismissing them as "flat-earthers".

NW: I get that. But you can't change the physical facts.

BB: Let me be clear: I agree, if you have a different thought or feeling, your brain chemistry will change in alliance with that thought or feeling. But you can also understand why antipsychiatry folk largely steer clear of that kind of analysis.

NW: It's a problem when people in antipsychiatry deny the neurodiversity involved in madness.

BB: Perhaps, but you can understand how this happens; there is a threat here that it will bring back the bogus causal claims. You know, there are parts of the mad movement that cannot be threatened even when it comes to alleged chemical imbalances. For unlike the antipsychiatry movement, they say: It is irrelevant to us whether or not our brains are different than so-called normals. It is irrelevant whether or not we have chemical imbalances. It is irrelevant because all there is is diversity.

NW: And that's my position as well.

BB: I know that, but given this position within the mad movement, you can see why its adherents can ally more easily with the neurodiversity movement than the antipsychiatry movement can. That said, I would like to see an alliance of all these movements.

NW: As would I. You know, when I got into the autistic movement, I saw the value of the word "neurodiversity". And so I became a theorist who helps define the concept and the paradigm. Now the word rang true to me at the time; nonetheless, hearing how some of the mad pride activists take exception to it, also given my knowledge of how autism gets essentialized as neurobiological, I am also feeling that there are flaws with the word.

BB: Moreover, there are both radical and far-from-radical neurodiversity theorizing.

NW:	Absolutely. So while I am happy with the work that I have done in terms of the neurodiversity paradigm, that is not where my work is now going.
BB:	Where are you going, Nick?
NW:	My focus is on cognitive liberty.
BB:	Which is a terrific concept around which all these related movements could easily unite. People have to be allowed to think in the ways that they do.
NW:	Yes, we all have cognitive liberty as a bottom line. So that is increasingly what I am presenting.
BB:	A very helpful direction. And there would be little or no tension between our respective movements when it comes to this concept.
NW:	And in that sense I am willing to embrace. . .
BB:	(laughing) Being a cognitive liberty activist?
NW:	Yes. Particularly in terms of spreading that concept. I would like to help people from all these related movements unite under the banner of cognitive liberty.
BB:	A direction in which I see real promise. That said, before we end, is there any question that you would like to answer that I haven't asked?
NW:	Well, I'd like to address what there is beyond general theory, fighting, and activism.
BB:	Sure. Are you referring here to the building of a better world?
NW:	Yes, because again, I am not in a fight here.
BB:	Rather, you are in the process of constructing a new way of being.
NW:	Yes, I am building something because, as I see it, right now on top of the power they wield, there is a marked advantage that the forces of psychiatry, psychology, and behaviorism have over us. Even though their solutions don't work and are abusive, they actually have things they call "solutions". So I want to personally go to building actual solutions.
BB:	So, for instance, you want ways to help people deal with the trauma in their lives?
NW:	Exactly, for a critical problem we are facing is that we have traumatized communities. Now for a lot of years, I was a person recovering from PTSD. But now I am largely recovered.
BB:	PTSD? Now that's a surprise! So you *use* the psychiatric term?
NW:	Yes, because we have to be able to deal with trauma.

BB:	You know, I write and teach extensively on trauma [see Burstow 2003, 2018], and I never use such terms.
NW:	How interesting! I should read your works.
BB:	Perhaps also the writing of other feminists who have likewise taken the lead on this issue [e.g., Brown, 1995]. That said, we can work with trauma more effectively if we don't buy into the psychiatric paradigm.
NW:	I don't want to buy into the psychiatric paradigm; nonetheless, there are lingering effects that abuse has.
BB:	Of course there are. And there is no problem whatever with you talking about this and using the word "trauma". On the other hand, there *is* a problem with you using the term "PTSD" or "Posttraumatic Stress Disorder". Insofar as you use such terms, you are calling people's natural responses to the terrible things that have happened to them a disorder.
NW:	Ah!
BB:	Trauma is a natural reaction which people have to terrible events or processes which they have undergone, and if we are to help and not hurt them further, we need to bear this reality firmly in mind. If someone is raped, say, being frightened is a natural reaction. And cutting themselves, by the same token, is a natural reaction that many to have to pain. A way of dealing with it.
NW:	Absolutely.
BB:	By contrast, what do psychiatric terms like PTSD do? They strip people of the context which makes their reactions natural. And then there is the intrusion that they invite. What do these terms invite in? Drugging, for example, because you have these disordered reactions and so forth.
NW:	I've not thought about that before.
BB:	It is part of the same paradigm shift. Bottom line: "The master's tools can never dismantle the master's house" [see Lorde 1984].
NW:	I totally agree. That acknowledged, to get back to my main point, we have these traumatized communities and they are playing out the effects of their trauma on how they deal with each other. And new generations are becoming traumatized.
BB:	Sure. And unless we interrupt it, the cycle of trauma continues.
NW:	Abuse by behaviorists, by psychologists, and by psychiatrists
BB:	And abuse by other traumatized people.

NW: So it is problematic when we are just "antipsychiatry" or "people defending autistic rights". The point here is that we are *fighting against* something but we are not *creating* anything.

BB: I acknowledge the validity of your critique. At the same time, I should point out that some of us who identify as antipsychiatry are also building. In this regard, you might want to read the last and largest chapter of my book *Psychiatry and the Business of Madness* [Burstow 2015], for it explicitly covers how to be helpful to traumatized people, how to address conflict, and how to build a better society.

NW: Wonderful! So I am interested in transformative practice. And I am particularly interested in building traditions of transformative practice that are mad, and queer, and neurodivergent. What I am grappling with is: How can we build a more accepting, more spiritual culture where we can be the best people that we can?

BB: A question and a direction that speaks to me. And on that note, Nick, thank you for this interview. And do keep being the enlightened visionary and builder that you are.

REFERENCES

Brown, L. (1995). Not outside the range: One woman's perspective. In C. Caruth (Ed.), *Trauma: Explorations in memory.* Baltimore: John Hoskins University Press.

Burstow, B. (2003). Toward a radical understanding of trauma work. *Violence Against Women, 10*(11), 1293–1317.

Burstow, B. (2015). *Psychiatry and the business of madness: An ethical and epistemological accounting.* New York: Palgrave Macmillan.

Burstow, B. (2018). *Teaching counterhegemonic trauma courses: A "kick-ass" way to be antipsychiatry.* Downloaded May 31, 2018 from https://breggin.com/bonnie-burstow/

Kuhn, T. (1962). *The structure of scientific revolutions.* Chicago: University of Chicago Press.

Lorde, A. (1984). *Sister outsider.* Berkeley: Crossing Press.

REPRESENTATIVE PUBLICATIONS OF NICK WALKER

Walker, N. (2013). *Throw away the master's tools: Liberating ourselves from the pathology paradigm.* Downloaded August 6, 2018 from http://neurocosmopolitanism.com/throw-away-the-masters-tools-liberating-ourselves-from-the-pathology-paradigm/

Walker, N. (2014a). *Neurodiversity: Some basic terms and definitions.* Downloaded August 6, 2018 from http://neurocosmopolitanism.com/neurodiversity-some-basic-terms-definitions/

Walker, N. (2014b). *Neurotypical psychotherapists & neurotypical clients.* Downloaded August 6, 2018 from http://neurocosmopolitanism.com/neurotypical-psychotherapists-and-neurodivergent-clients/

Walker, N. (2014c). *Neuroqueer: An introduction.* Downloaded August 6, 2014 from http://neurocosmopolitanism.com/neuroqueer-an-introduction/

Walker, N. (2015). What is autism? And this is autism. In M. Sutton (Ed.), *The real experts: Parents of autistic children.* Fort Worth: Autonomous Press.

Walker, N. (2016a). *Autism and the pathology paradigm.* Downloaded August 6, 2018 from http://neurocosmopolitanism.com/autism-and-the-pathology-paradigm/

Walker, N. (2016b). Kelly's blackbird. In M. S. Monje & N. I. Nicholson (Eds.), *The spoon knife anthology: Thoughts on compliance, defiance, and resistance.* Fort Worth: Neuroqueer Press.

Walker, N. (2017). Bianca and the Wu-Hernandez. In D. A. Ryskamp & S. Harvey (Eds.), *Spoon knife 2: Test chamber.* Fort Worth: NeuroQueer Books.

Walker, N. (2018a). In N. Walker & A. M. Reichart (Eds.), *Spoon knife 3: Incursions.* Fort Worth: NeuroQueer Books.

Walker, N. (2018b). Somatic and autistic embodiment. In D. H. Johnson (Ed.), *Diversity bodies, diversity practices: Toward an inclusive society.* Berkley: North Atlantic Books.

Nick's Added Comment

A term like "neurodiversity" might be useful to a given person or community, while others might be put off because they associate "neuro" with the false narratives about "brain diseases" and "chemical imbalances" that psychiatry uses to medicalize cognitive noncompliance. But those of us working for cognitive liberty must not allow ourselves to get caught up in conflicts over details of language and ideology, at the expense of forming empathic connections and working in solidarity toward shared goals.

All oppression and abuse of noncompliant body/minds, under the guise of "treatment", is part of the same overarching social paradigm. This is true whatever form the so-called treatment takes—institutionalization, forced drugging, electrocution, nonconsensual medical procedures, behaviorist compliance training (ABA), bleach enemas (that's a thing that's done to autistic children), or whatever the latest atrocity is. It's true whether the noncompliance that's being punished (oh, excuse me, I mean "treated") happens to take the form of madness, or autism, or queerness or gender nonconformity, or some combination of these.

A large-scale cultural shift toward greater cognitive liberty can only be effected through solidarity among the cognitively noncompliant. I offer "cognitively noncompliant" as a term to encompass all of us whose cognitive liberty is threatened by the paradigm of compulsory normativity of which all coercive "treatments" are manifestations. The spectrum of cognitive noncompliance encompasses all forms of queerness, neurodivergence, and madness.

Solidarity in cognitive noncompliance means that those who identify as mad, those who identify as autistic or otherwise neurodivergent, and those who identify as queer, all stop disavowing one another and throwing one another under the proverbial bus. It means mutual tolerance for the differences among us rather than squabbling over trivialities like our preferences in terminology. It means individuals making daily choices to put the goals of solidarity, compassion, and cognitive liberty above the temptation to get sucked down into the muck of "callout culture", petty one-upmanship, and the endless opportunities to take offense.

When we scorn each other and tear each other down over our differences, we subvert our higher goals. The dominant paradigm we purport to oppose is built on hostility toward difference. Reacting to our mutual differences from a position of hostility just perpetuates this paradigm (the master's tools will never dismantle the master's house). Effective noncompliance meets differences with love.

CHAPTER 11

Dialogue with Indigenous Leader and Psych Survivor Michael

This conversation is with one of my very favorite colleagues—Michael. Because of the need for anonymity, Michael is not using his official name, and for the same reason, no list of his publications follows.

A member of the Mi'kmaq nation, Michael is an Indigenous scholar committed to traditional ceremony. He is a university faculty member who teaches Indigenous Studies at one of the universities on Turtle Island. He is also a victim/survivor of the Sixties Scoop (a horrendous practice in the 1960s wherein Indigenous children in Canada and Mexico were stolen from their parents and then adopted out in the US). Michael is likewise a psychiatric survivor.

While I have known Michael for only a few years, the bond between us is palpable. That bond arises from a shared critique of psychiatry, from a commitment to Indigenous resurgence, though also from the fact that we both come from communities that have experienced genocide (in his case, Indigenous, and in my case, Jewish)—with both of us implicitly trusting in that connection.

BB: Michael, I am so delighted that you have joined this project. As you are particularly concerned about what psychiatry has done and continues to do to Indigenous people—and how could one not be?—how about we focus in on that? In one of our many exchanges over the last year, you said, "Psychiatry loves to target Indigenous people, label us crazy, and then incarcerate us." I couldn't agree more. Would you like to enlarge on that?

© The Author(s) 2019   149
B. Burstow, *The Revolt Against Psychiatry*,
https://doi.org/10.1007/978-3-030-23331-0_11

M: Absolutely. As Indigenous people, we are an easy group to target. Traditionally, we've had no voice. Personally, I was born when whatever the Indian agents said was law—you couldn't contest it. So the power was there. Let me add, what happened and what continues to happen to us, isn't done by accident. It is done by design. The point is, subjecting people to psychiatry is an easy way to silence them. And once we are silenced, why should they listen to us about land claims or anything else?

BB: Absolutely. So would it be fair to say that like me, you see the psychiatrization of Indigenous people as essentially part of a colonial enterprise—this, irrespective of the fact the psychiatric establishment call this psychiatrization "help"?

M: Without question.

BB: Where not help but disempowerment is the goal?

M: Yes. And that happens both systemically and personally.

BB: Let's step for a moment into the personal. You know what has been done to Indigenous people as a scholar who analyses history, but you also know it on a far deeper level. Please say as much or as little as you like, but how would you feel about telling us what happened to you at the hands of psychiatry? A story, as I understand it, if we are to comprehend it properly, which dates back the Sixties Scoop.

M: Sure … You know, this is the first time I've told this story.

BB: The story about being psychiatrized?

M: Yes.

BB: I didn't realize. Michael, do you want to take a minute here?

M: No, it actually feels good to be saying something. For things to change, it is critical for our stories to come out. So here goes: I was adopted during the Sixties Scoop. Well, what happened was against my parents' wishes. So I don't know how you want to call it—do I dare call it kidnapping? "Adoption" sounds too benign.

BB: Far too benign. Yes, this was a kidnapping. As part of one of the great crimes of history, you were stolen from your parents and your community, leaving both you and your people bereft.

M: Thank you for that. And you know, the fear I showed just now about using the accurate word "kidnapping", this fear is something instilled in those of us who are Indigenous. We are taught that these profound interferences were acts of kindness and that we'd better go along with this depiction. They weren't.

BB: Sure not.

M: No one, absolutely no one has the right to remove children when they are not in harm's way. And we weren't. Now the reason why we were removed and taken across the border to the United States was only because we were First Nations people. It was to assimilate us and to break the community. Many of the older people on the reserve point to this as one of two pivotal moments that led people in the community to begin drinking. The first time was in 1929 when the residential schools began.

BB: Not coincidentally, if I might say this, both actions involving the stealing of children and the profound injury thereby done not only to the child but to the community. Something I have learnt from Indigenous leaders who were kind enough to mentor me, you remove a child from a community as holistic and child-centered as Indigenous communities are, and both the child and the community is lost.

M: Precisely. And there was nothing our parents could do. Now for me, I grew up not knowing my family. I was adopted out in the US. I remember very little of this. Though even to this day, I regularly have nightmares about being kidnapped. It's very strange. Whenever I am in unfamiliar surroundings, I suddenly become afraid. And I have to make sure the door is locked. Say I am lying down. Suddenly with nothing having led to this, I get up and check to ensure sure that the door's locked. I am not sure why.

BB: I am so sorry about what happened to you, Michael. As for why you have to check if the door is locked, if I might hazard a guess, I suspect for similar reasons that decades after the Holocaust ended, survivors found themselves sleeping with their boots on. In these acts that seem strange, in these responses that seem out of keeping, we get a glimpse into the enormity of the trauma caused.

M: Yes.

BB: So, you were kidnapped and ended up in a settler family in the States and thankfully, that family, as it happened, was a loving family.

M: It was.

BB: None of which obliterates the fact that your life was turned upside-down and you were traumatized. And then at some point, you ended up directly falling prey to psychiatry. How did that happen? And what were the consequences?

M: On top of the terror that would creep upon me and the general sense of being vulnerable, I identify as two-spirited; I was growing up in the 1970s, and there just wasn't a place for me to understand what was going on with me or to talk about it. Everything outside of me was telling me that how I was feeling was wrong. That I could change if I prayed. Anyway, I thought that I was bad. I attempted suicide at age 16. I was taken to hospital and put in the care of a psychiatrist almost immediately. Now on my birth certificate, it said, "Red". And when the psychiatrist saw that, he began to ask me about my First Nations background. I told him I don't know where I'm from. Anyway, instead of probing this enigma, he almost immediately put me on antipsychotics.

BB: As if the problem facing you could be put down a chemical imbalance and/or bad genes? Colonialism at its most insidious.

M: Yes. And the experience that followed is something that I will never forget. It was like being stuck in a nightmare. Like the pictures in Alice in Wonderland. Everything became distorted and strange. And this went on a long time.

BB: Sounds to me like a new assault, yet another replacement of real identity—two spirited Indigenous—with a colonized identity—mentally ill person—and a compounding of the trauma.

M: Yes, that rings true to me. Now fortunately, deep down I knew that the only way to get better is to leave. Unfortunately, though, when I tried to, staff dragged me back and tied me to my bed. At any rate, though I was only 16, it did sink in that the thing wrong with me was the medication. Fortunately, my family knew it too, but it took them awhile to get me out. The hospital of course justified their actions on the grounds that I was a danger to myself.

BB: And so no one said: "You're having an identity crisis in part because you are a stolen child who have been wrenched from your community."

M: No, they just saw me as ill and in need of medication.

BB: In the process, completely ignoring the colonial history. Now eventually, you did go out…

M: And my parents helped me get off the drugs.

BB: Thank God you had sensible and kind adoptive parents. Nonetheless, in your story lies a window onto the brutality reality of settler colonialism.

M: That's my sense too. Bonnie, could you say more about what you are seeing?

BB: You were a kid and you were stolen from your people. And the problems that you inevitably ended up facing as a result such as not knowing who you are and not seeming to fit were subsequently treated as a medical disorder with drugs entering in to control you. And to expand the focus here, when we look at what has happened to Indigenous people, what we see is a genocidal practice, then psychiatry enters in and further damages the same population by labeling, drugging, and incarcerating, in essence, continuing the genocide.

M: That's it.

BB: Personally, what I am seeing right now—and I wonder if you could comment on it—is psychiatry today has targeted the Indigenous community as the population most in need of "psychiatric services", positioning this as help when what is happening is actually an extension of colonialism. In the process, many psychiatric institutions are hiring indigenous workers, calling this a meeting of communities when to me, it looks more like cooptation. I know that I've said a mouthful here. But could you comment?

M: The question is: *Who* are they hiring? Do the Indigenous people being hired know the history of their nations? Are they grounded in ceremonial life? Do they see the bigger picture? Do they understand that subjection to psychiatry is itself part of genocide? To explain what I am getting at here, the residential schools, the Sixties Scoop, psychiatrization, all this is about keeping people in a state where they can't think. And we see signs of the invasion everywhere. You know, I just visited my reserve last week. What a mess it was! There is a full-time doctor there doing nothing but prescribing psychiatric drugs. And that makes no sense. There never was a doctor present when people were sick from *real* diseases. Not even a dentist.

BB: A very telling contradiction! You know, what I see as apropos here, throughout the world right now there is a movement called the Movement for Global Mental Health. And what they do is not dissimilar. They target oppressed colonized communities throughout the world for "special psychiatric help". Psychiatrists go into religious spaces more or less hand-in-hand with the local healers who perform local religious ceremonies while the medical doctor dispenses psychiatric drugs to everyone [for further details, see Chap. 14]. And herein lies not only further colonization but the cooptation of the community in the process.

M: Not my sense of what we need. What we need is to be listened to and to have our records open; we need something done about land claims; we need promises honored—that's what we need—not drugs. The psychiatrization keeps us from thinking. And the inroads made into the Indigenous community keeps us from organizing. And once again, getting us all on drugs doesn't happen by accident. It is happening by design. Another thing: Our collective consciousness is our ceremony. And that's where we really need to go. I have already shared with you my first encounter with psychiatry. Let me share my second: It happened here in Toronto at St. Michaels Hospital. And this again had to do with being two-spirited. A relationship of mine had just ended and once again I fell into thinking that my two-spirited life was just wrong. And like people suggested, I prayed, but of course nothing changed. To make a long story short, I again attempted suicide. And again I was taken to hospital. And again, I was put on antipsychotics. Anyway, I remember the staff person coming to talk to me and saying, "Oh, so you're First Nations.. . That's interesting." That always stuck with me. Why did he say that? What did he think that had to do with what happened?

BB: Correct me if I am wrong here, Michael, but my guess is that you are suggesting that his comment arose not from his taking seriously the role of colonization, but rather from his negative stereotypes about Indigenous people?

M: Precisely. Anyway, I kept insisting that I wanted to go home. And he said, no you're not well and so we have to watch you. They kept observing me. They isolated me. They wouldn't even let me make a phone call. Finally, some people from the Indigenous community visited me. And I connected up with First Nations Support Services. To cut to the chase, I finally got out and sought out Indigenous people who led me through a four-day fast. I partook of ceremony, and I had a traditional feast. And I took part in a talking circle. And this was the beginning of my ceremonial journey. And that's what helped me be me. That's what healed me. To be clear, those four days helped me more than anything else in my entire life.

11 DIALOGUE WITH INDIGENOUS LEADER AND PSYCH SURVIVOR MICHAEL   155

BB: I can only imagine what a relief it was. And *of course*, it helped, because it was a critical part of what you needed. If I might hazard a guess, this is part of what your spirit longed for. You didn't need psychiatry interfering with you. And how wonderful you understood that!

M: Psychiatry just interferes with us. It always has.

BB: That said, I wonder if you could touch just briefly on the history of psychiatry's treatment of Indigenous people. A place that might be good to begin is the legendary and infamous Hiawatha Asylum for Insane Indians.

M: Actually, I know nothing except the name and that it was a bad place. I suspect you've been researching this. Bonnie, could you tell me more about it?

BB: You sure you want me to use up your time going into this?

M: A hundred per cent sure.

BB: Historically, this was one of two major institutions in the US created to "serve" what was called "insane Indians". Behind this facade of help lies the project of colonization. The white establishment was intent on stealing land and children. And basically, any Indigenous person who posed a problem for the white establishment as it carried out its design was at risk of being labeled insane and incarcerated here. The institution opened its doors in 1899 and continued for decades. And something that may hold special meaning for you because of your own history, one of the many reasons people were placed here is that they were upset and complained about having their children removed from them.

M: That was the reason for being locked up?

BB: I am afraid so. The control here of a despised community is absolutely naked. You steal children, calling it for their own good. And then if the parents left bereft in the now shattered community complain, you steal them also, invalidating them in the process with the label "insane" and in essence, rendering resistance impossible.

M·   Oh my! And what happened to these people?

BB: The people so apprehended were isolated from everyone, often chained to the floor and left there for decades. The decision was made that they be sterilized so that they could not pass on the insanity—as I see it, with this interpretation and agenda being part and parcel of the eugenics movement in which psychiatry was intrinsically involved [for this connection, see Burstow 2015]—but

156 B. BURSTOW

they had no one to sterilize these people and so they just kept them locked up so that they could not procreate and thereby not pass on the putative insanity. Eventually after many decades, it was acknowledged that none of these people had ever been "insane", and the institution itself was shut down. So they opened the doors and let people go—broken and forlorn. Well, the few who were left, for hoards of hapless Indigenous inmates had already died and had been buried on the grounds. The epilogue to this story? After the structure had been razed to the ground, they built a modern golf course over the remains of the Indigenous people buried there. So just as the population was horrifically oppressed in life, they were further oppressed and cheated in death [for this and further details on this frightening piece of history, see Yellow Bird (n.d.)]

M: Unbelievable! Words fail me!

BB: Words fail me also. That said, there is a symbol here of incredible power. And there is a history here of mammoth abuse that likewise cries out for reparations. Michael, do you see this as possible site for social action?

M: Of course. Would they do this to any other race of people?

BB: My own sense? Yes and no. What has happened to Black people at the hands of psychiatry is likewise a horror show. As I discuss in my book *Psychiatry and the Business of Madness* (Burstow 2015) incredible and pervasive racism is built into the very fabric of psychiatry.

M: Let me rephrase. Would they do this to white people? No.

BB: Agreed. Psychiatry is vile to everyone but racialized people are treated far worse on the basis of bogus biological theories of inferiority and the psychiatrization of people of color is itself part of larger societal design.

M: Yes.

BB: Which brings us to the question of resistance. You have started to think of getting involved on a political level with combating psychiatry. And there are many ways to resist. My own sense is that every time you as a spiritual leader reinstate traditional ceremony, you are resisting—and I very much respect that. When you left St Michael's Hospital and sought out traditional healers, this in itself is resistance. And this is something that that those of us who are settlers have no place in whatever. That said, do you see a space to also work with certain settlers here—and of course I mean ones into resistance? While I realize that I am asking a complicated question, can you imagine some kind or alliance between Indigenous people committed to Indigenous resurgence and the antipsychiatry movement?

M: Absolutely.

BB: If you think the antipsychiatry movement might have a role to play here, what do you think that role may look like?

M: Supporting us in our efforts to restore a ceremonial life. Supporting us in our emphasis on settling land claims. Making people aware.

BB: Including of the destructive role that psychiatry plays in the Indigenous world?

M: Absolutely.

BB: For us to be decent allies here, I also think it's imperative for the antipsychiatry movement more generally to expand to centrally include Indigenous issues. Is this a direction that you can imagine yourself taking a lead with respect to? And how do you see that happening?

M: Joining with antipsychiatry can only benefit us. And it is not "if" we can. It is "when" we can and hammering out how.

BB: Just off the top of my head, Michael, one route might be—and to be clear, I suspect there are lots of paths—is Indigenous leaders like yourself who have an explicitly Indigenous analysis coming into general antipsychiatry groups or inviting us to enter your space and teaching everyone what *has happened* to Indigenous people and community, what *is happening,* and how to be allies. Helping us integrate the Indigenous story/stories more fully, helping us to understand aspects that we need to understand better and be ready to act on them, while of course taking the lead from the Indigenous communities themselves. Do you see that as one kind of inroad that might be made?

M: For sure. This would help disseminate information. The telling of our stories that would be involved. This would bring us obvious allies. And telling others what happened to us, this is a route to healing.

BB: You know, again, off the top of my head, and once again I am only just brainstorming now, how about expanding on a direction that has always been pivotal in both the psychiatric survivor community and the Indigenous community—the giving of testimony? I think there may be some kind of a match, albeit clearly there are differences too—between psychiatric survivors needing to tell their story and Indigenous people needing to tell their stories. Again, I am just speculating here: But what if Indigenous leaders like yourself joined forces with groups like Coalition Against Psychiatric Assault to set up public hearings, wherein Indigenous people harmed by psychiatry could come bear testimony? What if we looked into organizing an Indigenous speak-out somewhere like Toronto City Hall? There would the sheer power of the live testimony. There would be the triumph of individually and collectively bearing witness. And besides the immediacy, the testimony could be put on the internet.

M: What a fantastic thing to do!

BB: Needless to say, the antipsychiatry movement would have to take direction from Indigenous spiritual leaders here, with traditional healing ceremony necessarily being centrally involved.

M: Ceremony, absolutely.

BB: Do think about whether or not you want to continue to explore this idea and do let me know about other possible initiatives that occur to you. That said, we are coming to the end of our discussion today. Michael, thank you so much for taking part in this dialogical interview, for being part of this project, for thinking together with me, for your wisdom, and for your story.

M: No, my friend, thank-*you*.

REFERENCES

Burstow, B. (2015). *Psychiatry and the business of madness.* New York: Palgrave Macmillan.

Yellow Bird, Pemima. (n.d.). *Wild Indians: Native perspectives on the Hiawatha Asylum for Insane Indians.* Downloaded February 10, 2017 from https://power2u.org/wild-indians-native-perspectives-on-the-hiawatha-asylum-for-insane-indians-by-pemima-yellow-bird/

CHAPTER 12

"This Is Not a Time to Lie Low": Dialogue with International Lawyer, Survivor, and Human Rights Advocate Tina Minkowitz

Tina Minkowitz is a human rights lawyer and a survivor of forced psychiatric interventions. She is founder and president of the Center for the Human Rights of Users and Survivors of Psychiatry (http://www.chrusp.org), a user/survivor-led human rights organization with Special Consultative Status with the UN Economic and Social Council (UN ECOSOC). Current projects of hers include The Absolute Prohibition Campaign (http://absoluteprohibition.org) and the Convention on the Rights of Persons with Disabilities (CRPD) course taught from the survivor of psychiatry perspective (http://crpdcourse.org). Previously, she served the World Network of Users and Survivors of Psychiatry (http://wnusp.wordpress.com), leading its work in the drafting and negotiation of the CRPD (see https://www.un.org/development/desa/disabilities/convention-on-the-rights-of-persons-with-disabilities.html), which has brought about a revolution in international human rights law. The CRPD requires ratifying state parties to abolish forced interventions and deprivation of liberty in mental health settings and to replace substitute decision-making with universal adult legal capacity and non-coercive support. Tina has also published extensively.

Tina and I met when I became involved in an initiative of hers—The Campaign to Support the CRPD Absolute Prohibition of Forced Treatment and Commitment (http://absoluteprohibition.org). Correspondingly, she has contributed to two of my books.

© The Author(s) 2019
B. Burstow, *The Revolt Against Psychiatry*,
https://doi.org/10.1007/978-3-030-23331-0_12

159

BB: Tina, how about we zero in on the CRPD [Convention on the Rights of Persons with Disabilities]? As a lawyer and a survivor, you were key in ensuring the explicit inclusion of psychiatric survivor issues in this convention. To highlight a few of the important articles for readers less familiar with the Convention, while of all the articles are important, absolutely pivotal is 12, 14, and 4.

TM: I see 12 and 14 as the most important; 4.3 is likewise significant for it obliges government to actively consult people with disabilities through their representative organizations. Also other parts of article 4 require governments to abolish discriminatory laws.

BB: Which is huge. And article 12 is nothing short of revolutionary for it mandates an absolute presumption of capacity—period—correct?

TM: What's new about the presumption of capacity in article 12 is that it's an *irrebuttable* presumption. Now people might say, "The capacity legislation in my country has the presumption of legal capacity." However, that is generally "a *rebuttable* presumption"— that is, you're presumed to have legal capacity until your status is challenged, whereas the presumed capacity spelt out in the CRPD can never be denied or taken away.

BB: Which renders the psychiatrist's pronouncements about a person's legal capacity and the Draconian procedures for "determining" it utterly irrelevant.

TM: Exactly.

BB: And the significance of this for the psych survivor population is that no one can lock them up against their will or subject them to any "treatment" they don't want.

TM: Correct.

BB: So this is a fundamental paradigm shift.

TM: It is. Article 12 is the center of "the paradigm shift", but article 14, which prohibits the deprivation of liberty based on disability, is also crucial because locking people up derives from the state's power to establish what constitutes lawful detention. Likewise critical is article 25, which spells out the right to free and informed consent on an equal basis with others in health care because it helps us determine how article 12 is interpreted. Article 12 guarantees legal capacity "in all aspects of life"—the right to decide about *everything* pertaining to our own lives—which logically includes the decision to take or refuse "medication", where to live.

Having the right to free and informed consent explicitly mentioned gave us a textual basis to insist on the right to refuse treatment. One of the distinctions instrumental in how we went about the framing was to say: Sometimes people want support in making their decisions or understanding information, which is fine, and indeed states should be required to provide support, but you cannot actually remove people's right to make their own decisions. Being able to frame the issue that way was faithful to our own instincts and positions and was also critical in gaining the approval of the states that negotiated the treaty. We're not saying that no one ever needs support. What we're saying is that people have the right to decide for themselves if they want support and if so, what kind.

BB: A terrific move forward. On another level which is likewise exciting, what we're witnessing here is the problematic and age-old relationship between the state and psychiatry beginning to be severed.

TM: Yes. How psychiatry is able to operate as it does is through the power given it in legislation like the mental health acts and the capacity laws. What states have been doing is delegating to psychiatry the power of lawful detention and the power to act on people's bodies against their will. And we have argued to a degree successfully that forced psychiatric intervention amounts to torture. Under human rights laws and under international law generally, the state is responsible for ensuring that unlawful detention isn't practiced. And the CRPD specifies that detention based on disability is unlawful under international law. Correspondingly, it obliges states to remove this power from psychiatry. I think the power of detention is crucial because if they don't have the power to lock you up, they can't get you into a place where they can subject you to such interventions as forced drugging.

BB: I think you're slightly overstating what removing the power to forcibly detain single-handedly accomplishes. Even without detaining you, equipped with today's long-acting drugs, they could just track you down, grab you, and inject you—and you'd be stuck with the effect for months.

TM: That's true at the present time; however historically, forced drugging started in places of detention and detention is still used as a threat to enforce compliance in many outpatient commitment

162   B. BURSTOW

laws. In any case, that part is also covered because of the irrefutable presumption of capacity and the right to free and informed consent. The crucial thing will be how states put this into practice and how the various mental health systems respond to it. As you said, severing the relationship between the state and psychiatry is pivotal.

BB: And really, the state has made psychiatry worse and in turn, psychiatry makes the state worse.

TM: Yes.

BB: Let me go back to something you said earlier because there's an unfortunate wrinkle in all of this. Just like all current mental health laws, the CRPD employs the concept of "free and informed consent". That concept begs the question given that we know that the "information" that psychiatry provides is woefully inaccurate. How has the UN responded to this very obvious wrinkle—if at all?

TM: I don't know if that particular issue has been presented to the CRPD committee yet. The Special Rapporteur on Torture in his 2008 report specified what information was required for informed consent to electroshock, based on information that we provided to him. The CRPD Committee could similarly address this if information is provided to them about psychiatric drugs, but they have not yet gone into that level of detail.

BB: But you can see that the paradigm shift is much less substantial if psychiatry can still lure people into believing their misrepresentations and if, as a result, 90% of the people taking the "treatments" now continue to take them. That rather makes a mockery of the "informed" part of free and *informed* consent.

TM: Of course the aspect of "informed" consent has to be developed not only in disability nondiscrimination law but in human rights law as a whole. CRPD is a starting point but cannot do it all.

BB: Right. And an important starting point, though this is far from a minor issue.

TM: Agreed. The CRPD is based in the social model of disability. However, because we've been half in and half out of a disability framework, the situation is complicated.

BB: By "we" you mean?

TM: Psychiatric survivors.

BB: As I see it, the use of the word "disability" came in with the incorporation of disability into the definition of "mental disorder" in the opening pages of DSM-III-R [Diagnostic and Statistical Manual of Mental Disorders—Third Edition]. Then survivors accepted it because it proved useful when demanding rights.

TM: I was not aware of the word "disability" coming with the DSM. Many of us also accepted it because it is an accurate way to describe the discrimination we face, and this, I believe, has been the crux element in why the CRPD succeeded when earlier attempts at legal doctrine to abolish forced psychiatry failed. As I see it, it's useful also because of how the movement has developed. We had a split between "consumers" and "survivors". There are people who never want any part of psychiatry ever again, or any kind of services. Then there are people who ended up in psychiatry because they wanted some kind of support—they just didn't want to be tortured. And the concept of disability allows us to say, you have rights irrespective of whether or not you think there's something you need help with. And I see the social and the non-discrimination model of disability which the CRPD has put forward as unifying these different parts of the community. And then of course there are activists and thinkers in the global south who mainly see psychiatry as a western colonial imposition.

BB: Which it surely is.

TM: Absolutely. So they want a concept that they can relate to and that at the same time does not relate them to psychiatry. Which I see as a progressive move.

BB: Interesting and important. This said, how about we turn to what's actually happening on the ground? Now to the best of my knowledge, states which have signed and ratified the CRPD are obliged to repeal their mental health legislation, get rid of their locked wards, and to inform inmates that they are free to go. Question: Has a single country done that?

TM: Not that I know of. There are countries that never had mental health laws to begin with, albeit the practices are there.

BB. Okay, however it is happening, is anyone complying with the CRPD in any formidable way?

TM: There's been a few attempts, with no clear outcomes yet on a national level. One thing that I can tell you that is promising, the World Health Organization has withdrawn its earlier guidance telling states to enact mental health laws and instead is now providing training on how to transform mental health service based on what

164 B. BURSTOW

they are calling a recovery model. It is flawed but I honor their attempt to envision CRPD-compliant mental health policy. And the message is in the CRPD portion is loud and clear: You shouldn't be doing things to people against their will.

BB: All good, but at the same time the World Health Organization is pushing "global mental health", which is as colonizing as you can get [for details, see Chap. 14].

TM: There are different parts of the World Health Organization and I find the people doing this training sincere. They actually want to work for the abolition of force, which for them means promoting some version of the CRPD paradigm.

BB: Gotchya. And yes, that's promising. That said, in the end, another snaggle is that for good or for ill, the UN has no real power. Anyone can ignore any of its rulings.

TM: That's true.

BB: I know in Ontario, lawyers often laugh when the CRPD is brought up, for they are well aware it's not the law of the land and as far as they can see, it never will be. You see the problem.

TM: In BC [British Columbia, Canada's western-most province], which has the worst mental health legislation in Canada, lawyers are drawing on the CRPD in their challenge to the provincial mental health act.

BB: Which is great, Tina. At the same time, I cannot but ask: Are they getting any buy-in here from the judiciary?

TM: I don't think the suit has progressed yet.

BB: B.C. aside, has there ever been a suit in any country that has drawn on the CRPD and won?

TM: No, nobody has sued and won yet in cases of forced psychiatry. There is a judge in the US who on her own initiative used Article 12 to justify the recognition of supported decision-making as an alternative to guardianship.

BB: Yes, I heard about that, and that for sure is good news. But we still have to wait and see how this hypothetical possibility plays out with respect to the use of force. Now if the judiciary generally started recognizing the CRPD, of course—"whole new ballgame".

TM: The Working Group on Arbitrary Detention has called on courts to enforce the prohibition against disability-based detention. In other words, courts as a branch of the state can take on their own

12 "THIS IS NOT A TIME TO LIE LOW": DIALOGUE WITH INTERNATIONAL...   165

responsibility to comply with international law. And to the extent that there can be promotional activities that reach judges...

BB: That would be helpful?

TM: Yes. Countries differ on how they treat international law. In some countries you could go into the court simply with Article 12 and say, "My rights are being violated", and where the judge would have to take that into account. In others, no. Also countries adopt different doctrines and practices to circumvent international law.

BB: Agreed. Canada is an example. The ratification by Canada is a joke. What Canada says is "We are complying but *with this reservation—* our substitute decision-making counts", even though UN been very clear that it *does not count.*

TM: Indeed, and that's where advocacy comes in. In the Concluding Observations the CRPD Committee gave to Canada, they explicitly stipulated that the reservation is not permissible. It's an advocacy point.

BB: Which brings us back to what the judiciary does, right?

TM: There are many different avenues through which change could happen. There's the judiciary, there's the legislative route, as in repealing the mental health law. But it would take a lot of political mobilization.

BB: And you see different possible routes in different countries?

TM: Yes. Nonetheless, the dominant trend right now is to co-opt while side-stepping the paradigm shift. To give you an example of what I'm talking about, several countries are enacting legislation which include substitute decision-making *alongside* supported decision-making.

BB: So they are citing the CRPD while in direct violation of it? Making it look like they're complying when they aren't?

TM: Exactly. And none of the "reforms" currently under way involve eliminating the mental health laws. In one country—Peru—they briefly enacted a mental health law and repealed it after the CRPD committee so recommended. A legal capacity reform was proposed in the parliament, that, if enacted, would comply with the CRPD and probably eliminate any remaining basis for forced treatment or detention in a mental health context; however, the legislation stalled.

BB: And that elimination is a bottom line requirement—is what makes the CRPD the breakthrough that it is.

TM: Absolutely. What complicates matters further, cooptation politics that are familiar to all of us have been playing out within the international disability community and among legal scholars in the field. Shortly after the CRPD entry into force, I was at a meeting convened by the Open Society Institute [an organization that does a lot of funding in the disability community]. They had gathered together people they considered international experts on Article 12—and I was among them. One of the questions raised was whether to incorporate the issue of mental health laws and the abolition of forced treatment into the reform of legal capacity. And of course, that's precisely what I was advocating for. However, not a single other person in the room agreed with me—and that includes two other individuals identified with the user/survivor movement. This goes beyond questions of strategy. This is a question of basic principles. By the same token, some time after the CRPD was agreed to, a law reform took place in India and it is only after considerable advocacy occurred that the drafters even proposed to put in something about ending psychiatric detention—a provision on phasing it out, rather than outright elimination—and even that provision was removed from the final version of the law enacted. Meanwhile, India introduced a new mental health law which in essence continued "the same old thing"—forced treatment and detention.

BB: So they keep recreating the problem?

TM: Yes. I believe at this point that a new round of militancy needs to happen.

BB: Gotchya, because you're losing ground right now.

TM: We keep gaining and losing at the same time. I have comrades in Korea, in Norway, and in Chile, and in many other countries who are doing what they can to advocate for *real abolition.*

BB: By "abolition", you mean abolition of forced treatment and forced detention?

TM: Yes.

BB: You know, Tina, it's interesting. We both of us employ the word "abolition" and while we have something different in mind by the word, what I have in mind incorporates what you have in mind, which I suspect is why we're able to ally so readily.

TM: Bonnie, I'd be interested to hear what *you* have in mind. I suspect I'd agree with it also.

12 "THIS IS NOT A TIME TO LIE LOW": DIALOGUE WITH INTERNATIONAL... 167

BB: Well, in a nutshell, it's not just psychiatry's use of force but institutional psychiatry itself that I am looking to abolish.

TM: And concretely, what would that look like?

BB: Not only would it have no state power, it would not be propped up in any way by the state. Not stated funded, not state promoted. Not officially recognized as a "medical" discipline.

TM: While you're at it, you have to get rid of the whole notion of hegemony in the area of psychology and so forth.

BB: Absolutely, but you can't abolish an idea. So it's not the *notion of* hegemony, let me suggest, but the practices *embedded in it and that give rise to* hegemony that you need to get rid of.

TM: Yes, I am thinking about practices. The "mental health system" as a whole is problematic.

BB: Yes, in essence, it boils down to rule by the psy disciplines.

TM: Right.

BB: More generally, my own sense is that help should be arising from and be vested in the community at large. We should be trying to get away from the paradigm of professionals and experts. Bottom line—as long as we are stressing professional approaches, we will have power-over and we will have hegemony.

TM: Exactly. I agree.

BB: The two of us overlap more than I realized. That acknowledged, how about we shift into the personal? Tina, could you say something about how you came to be a lawyer fighting in this area—also what this means to you personally?

TM: Actually, that's a fascinating story. In some ways, I "fell into it". I was "locked up in psychiatry" when I was 18. About a month after I was released, I had this curious dream in which I saw myself as a lawyer.

BB: Wow!

TM: A few years later, at loose ends, I decided to enter law school. What happened is not as straight forward as you might imagine. For various reasons including contradictions between what I was hearing and what I'd experienced at the hands of the law when "locked up in psychiatry"—I decided that I didn't want to be a lawyer after all. About six months before I would have finished, I quit law school.

BB: I had no idea.

TM: While I did many things that interested me and had other jobs, the thought of what being a lawyer might open up kept coming back

168   B. BURSTOW

to haunt me. Finally, I decided: I need to go back and finish, to see what that would open up. So much time had passed, I was faced with starting all over, which I did.

BB: A truly courageous move, and if I might say so, one from which the world has benefited.

TM: I also decided to handle law school differently this time around. Not just to prepare for exams but to *really study*. So I went to CUNY Law School, whose motto is "Law in the Service of Human Needs". I had already been in touch with the Disability Rights Movement. I studied disability law and human rights law and for my third year, I did clinical work in the Women's International Human Rights Law Clinic.

BB: And in the process, you ended up venturing further and further into international law?

TM: Precisely. And I began thinking seriously about how to apply the principle of disability non-discrimination in international law to address psychiatric oppression.

BB: Now I'm just guessing here, but did you also start forming survivor groups?

TM: I tried to form a group in law school, but it wasn't possible. I did, though, have long-standing connections with survivor groups. Starting way back in 1978, I connected with the movement, and I was a member of Project Release [a New York group]. Later, I had joined WNUSP [The World Network of Users and Survivors of Psychiatry]—an organization that aims to represent users and survivors of psychiatry worldwide.

BB: A very formidable movement group which, with your help, was to eventually capture the ear of the UN.

TM: What happened is in 2001, I both graduated from law school and started hearing about this new UN convention people were going to start working on.

BB: The CRPD?

TM: Yes, and I heard that the group Mental Disability Rights International was saying things like: Let's keep a low profile. We just need to work for a strong non-discrimination clause and that will allow us to eventually challenge forced psychiatry. And I thought, no, this is our chance to make psychiatric survivor issues explicit. This is our chance to be heard by the international community in a forum that is dedicated to an outcome dealing with

12 "THIS IS NOT A TIME TO LIE LOW": DIALOGUE WITH INTERNATIONAL... 169

our human rights. This is not a time to lie low. This gives us the greatest leverage that we will ever have.

BB: Wonderful that you had the insight and seized the moment.

TM: There were several aspects to what happened, with luck itself playing a role. For instance, The World Network of Users and Survivors of Psychiatry had already been incorporated into the International Disability Alliance—a global alliance mainly of disabled people's organizations–and so it was already understood that the disability community is diverse and heterogenous, with different constituencies, each with its own perspective, and there was already a sense of what measures were important. I was able to ensure that issues related to the abolition of forced psychiatry were made explicit, framed in terms of disability nondiscrimination in basic human rights. I started talking about this in the movement before working on the Convention. I remember saying at a workshop in one of the conferences that the right to be free from forced interventions has to be seen as a core disability right on a par with reasonable accommodations and accessibility.

BB: Good for you and absolutely.

TM: And that is how I tried to frame it in the CRPD. And I pretty much succeeded.

BB: You surely did.

TM: We made valuable connections with other disability rights groups. We cultivated mutual support and found ways that our issues were linked in principle and practice.

BB: All of which allowed the CRPD as we know it to emerge. That said—and without question that's formidable—how is it that we are losing ground right now?

TM: We lack the degree of access and influence in international policymaking that we had in the context of the CRPD drafting and negotiation and the very early stages of interpretation. There are many reasons for this. Subsequent to the adoption of the Convention and its entry into force, solidarity among disability groups became weaker as we no longer had a common point of focus. Other interests came in—money interests. Academia. And of course, psychiatry and the mental health system started reacting, whereas they had not been present in the negotiations. My sense is there is a huge need right now to take a step further.

BB: And what would that further step be?

TM: Probably in the direction that you're calling abolition, Bonnie.

BB: This, I'd love to see! That said, there has to be huge opposition right now not only from psychiatry and the "mental health" system but the entire medical establishment. They have to be worried that their everyday approach to people labeled senile, for instance, may "all go out the window".

TM: The UN is starting to work on a convention on the rights of older persons.

BB: Which is absolutely great, but even before that comes about, the current provisions in the CRPD would require this population also to be treated as having "capacity".

TM: True, of course. I actually think it is the psychiatric survivor community that poses the greatest challenge to the medical establishment. We are the ones that reject the validity of their diagnoses. And we are the ones that challenge their hegemony in ways which go beyond the issue of state power.

BB: Absolutely. To how we understand being human. To how we understand society. And lest we forget even for a second, it is the people that society sees as "crazy" that the average person most fears and as a result, actually wants "under control".

TM: Right. Even in this major disability rights process, we remain very much marginalized and isolated. Our issues keep getting put back into the basket of "mental health and human rights". The context in which the UN itself currently is focusing on our issues, that is, is in seminars and conferences on "mental health and human rights". Which depoliticizes them utterly. Yes, we need to be changing the "mental health system" but that's not all we should be dealing with here. We need a fundamental shift—one that starts from a different vantagepoint.

BB: Absolutely.

TM: Along with my colleague Hege Orefellen in Norway, I have been promoting a reparations framework as a primary way for psych survivor issues to be dealt with. Forced psychiatry constitutes a system of widespread and grave human rights violations which the state has enabled. Under international law the state is responsible for making reparations at the individual level and also at the collective level. And this can include things like a public apology, memorials and histories, and most importantly, guarantees of non-repetition, which means ensuring that that these atrocities are stopped and do not happen again.

BB: Whether or not it has a ghost of a chance of gaining traction, an impressive move, that—for with this dimension on the table, the fact that we are talking about an actual oppression here becomes very clear.

TM: Exactly! Hege and her colleagues at We Shall Overcome [a Norwegian survivor organization] have just put reparations on the table in advocacy that may result in a recommendation to Norway by the CRPD Committee. This is exciting because it might actually gain traction now. And speaking to your comment that we are talking about an actual oppression here—one of the implications is that mental health professionals are sidelined instead of being in the center of the discussion.

BB: I couldn't agree more. While professionals can be included, professionals should not be at the center. *Survivors* should be at the center. And what needs to be taken in is that we are talking about dire transgressions which have been going on for centuries.

TM: When you think about survivor knowledge, there is just so much more that *could be* and *should be* happening. And why isn't it? One reason is cooptation, a perennial problem. Among other things, we have been marginalized by changes in the International Disability Alliance [IDA], which was taken over by staff, resulting in a centralization of power. IDA became a way for the UN to "manage" the international disability movement. Which is problematic for the disability movement as a whole but especially for us—though, the other side is, for some people in the user/survivor movement, it's also created opportunities to get training and to participate as trainers.

BB: Yeah, I do understand how this happens.

TM: To be fair, it has done some good, especially for people in the global south, but those gains come at a very hefty price. The price is the self-definition that our movement needs to have—one that's really independent from....

BB: Professionals?

TM: It's not necessarily mental health professions that are the problem this time. We also need to be independent of the influence of funders, other NGOs, and anyone with money and power that is working on our issues. There are survivors in the global south who

172   B. BURSTOW

would disagree with what I'm saying; from their perspective, they are self-determining. They don't want to be dictated to by survivors in the global north. And you know, about that, they're absolutely right.

BB: They surely are—which makes the way forward complicated to say the least. My guess is that survivors in the global south and survivors in the global north need to come together in dialogue.

TM: We have not been able to pull together when faced with difficult choices about relationships with other organizations. Then everyone develops their own relationships with outside partners.

BB: And would you say that this development is endangering the movement? Is making a unified approach almost impossible?

TM: It's hard to tell people not to take advantage of opportunities that come their way. And they are pursuing their own vision and focusing on what they see as most important. There is a movement emerging in all regions of the global south; and we all agree on the bottom line of no forced treatment and full human rights, not being relegated to service user status. So I see the potential for many things to develop in ways that will take us forward—even if I don't agree with all the ways people want to get there.

BB: All the more reason that there needs to be space for survivor-to-survivor and survivors/allies dialogue, which, of course would have to include efforts to decenter the global north within the movement.

TM: We surely need that and many of us actively work for it.

BB: All of which reminds me how very precarious our "best laid plans" are once we enter the public arena. And on that note, Tina, it's time for us to wrap up. *Mazel tov* on what you've been able to pull off to date! And good luck with the very real battles that lie ahead. Oh and do keep us posted.

TM: I will.

REPRESENTATIVE PUBLICATIONS OF TINA MINKOWITZ

Minkowitz, T. (2007). The United Nations convention on the rights of persons with disabilities and the right to be free from nonconsensual psychiatric interventions. *Syracuse Journal of International Law and Commerce, 34*(2), 405–428.

Minkowitz, T. (2010). *Norms and implementation of CRPD Article 12*. Downloaded August 24, 2018 from https://ssrn.com/abstract=2037452 or http://dx.doi.org/10.2139/ssrn.2037452

Minkowitz, T. (2012). *CRPD advocacy by the World Network of Users and Survivors of Psychiatry: The emergence of a user/survivor perspective in human rights.* Downloaded August 24, 2018 from https://ssrn.com/abstract=2326668 or https://doi.org/10.2139/ssrn.232Mi6668

Minkowitz, T. (2013). *We name it torture.* Downloaded August 24, 2018 from https://www.madinamerica.com/2013/06/we-name-it-torture/

Minkowitz, T. (2014a). *A response to a report by Juan Mendes, Special Rapporteur on Torture, dealing with torture in the context of healthcare, as it pertains to nonconsensual psychiatric interventions in Torture in Healthcare settings: Reflections on the Special Rapporteur on Torture's 2013 Thematic Report.* American University Center for Human Rights and Humanitarian Law Anti-Torture Initiative. https://www.academia.edu/27634155/A_response_to_the_report_by_Juan_E._M%C3%A9ndez_Special_Rapporteur_on_Torture_dealing_with_torture_in_the_context_of_healthcare_as_it_pertains_to_nonconsensual_psychiatric_interventions

Minkowitz, T. (2014b). *Rethinking criminal responsibility from a critical disability perspective: The abolition of insanity/incapacity acquittals and unfitness to plead, and beyond. Griffith Law Review, 23*(4), 434–466. https://doi.org/10.1080/10383441.2014.1013177.

Minkowitz, T. (2015a). *Meta-autonomy and meta-equality.* Downloaded August 24, 2018 from https://www.madinamerica.com/2015/09/meta-autonomy-and-meta-equality/

Minkowitz, T. (2015b). *What would CRPD-compliant legislation look like?* Downloaded August 24, 2018 from https://www.madinamerica.com/2015/05/what-would-crpd-compliant-mental-health-legislation-look-like/

Minkowitz, T. (2017a). *Free and Informed Consent and the Right to Refuse Treatment,' for ERC Voices Project at NUI Galway.* Video recording of panel: https://youtube/HMtwP5DLqEc and slides. Downloaded August 24, 2018 from https://www.youtube.com/watch?v=HMtwP5DLqEc&list=PLvKS9kpe3SYPAkFNESull duLXp9gknajx&index=2&t=0s

Minkowitz, T. (2017b). CRPD and transformative equality. *International Journal of Law in Context, 13*(1), 77–86.

Also see Author's SSRN page at page at. http://ssrn.com/author=1348856

TINA'S ADDED COMMENT

The genius of the CRPD for psychiatric survivors is that our rights are normalized and not set aside as an afterthought or a special case. We were uniquely positioned in that drafting process to make our human rights visible within the social model of disability and contribute to creating a complex, multidimensional legal doctrine of equality for people with all kinds of disabilities. We took a space that existed for us, but we took it in a way that the powers that be could not have expected. I do not know if the logic of non-discrimination persuaded them of our just cause, if it was simpler to support us with their fingers crossed behind their backs, or what combination of factors led to our qualified success in the treaty text, and the undoubted success with the treaty monitoring body and many though not all other UN entities. The national level presents undoubted difficulties, when we directly engage with political and legal processes that have maintained our oppression and now seek to involve them to overturn that oppression. What caught me by surprise were the attacks and marginalization from erstwhile allies and partners, who succumbed to negative propaganda against survivors of psychiatry that dare to take power for ourselves. Currently, we are lagging behind other disability rights constituencies in creating projects through a coherent global agenda with supportive partners (success defined in NGO terms), while doing sophisticated legal and political work to actively and continually challenge illegitimate power, using the new human rights tools we have created. Our messiness reflects the revolutionary character of our work, and the need to adapt and think creatively as the movement itself takes on the potential of the paradigm shift for freedom. It is *our* paradigm shift; we are the heavy lifters and continue to develop it in all the ways needed, to challenge the institutional power of mental health systems as well as that of the state.

CHAPTER 13

"I So Loved My Son that I Had to Promise Him that I'd Do Everything I Could": Dialogue with Mother and Archivist Julie Wood

Julie Wood is the mother of a psychiatrized child. She is also an archivist, an antipsychiatry activist, a researcher, and an educator. She is likewise a courageous human being. I will never forget the sheer admiration that I felt when I first encountered the following passage in an appeal she had lodged with the College of Physicians and Surgeons of Ontario with respect to their finding over a complaint she had lodged over the treatment of her son: "If John David was mentally ill, then so am I since we were temperamentally identical and it has never interfered with my ability to function at a high level" (for this and other statements by Julie in this appeal process, see Burstow 2015, Chapter 1). While I was acutely aware that these words would in no way lead the committee to rethink the utterly pathologizing narrative that they had constructed about John David, herein I saw a mother standing up for her son as only she could, and somewhere from deep in my soul, I found myself cheering, "Bravo!"

I first met Julie in 2010 when she turned up unexpectedly at a meeting of the Toronto activist group Coalition Against Psychiatric Assault. And we've been friends and co-activists together ever since.

BB: Julie, let me begin by thanking you for agreeing to be part of this project. I know that revisiting what you always end up having to revisit is never easy. That said, you came to critiquing psychiatry in

© The Author(s) 2019

B. Burstow, *The Revolt Against Psychiatry*,

https://doi.org/10.1007/978-3-030-23331-0_13

175

176 B. BURSTOW

a very different way than every single other person in this collection. How about telling us about that?

JW: Until ten years ago, I was one of those ordinary people who had no strong beliefs about psychiatry, no knowledge, and, as far as I could see, no reason whatever to worry about it. And it was the death of my son that changed everything. You see, my son [as a teenager] had taken a drug that was a stimulant—Dexedrine—for a friend of his had told him it helps you study—and he found a psychiatrist who was only too happy to prescribe it. And he took it in megadoses for several years.

BB: On the recommendation of the psychiatrist?

JW: Yes, and under the supposed supervision of the psychiatrist. Then John David told the psychiatrist he wanted to stop for he was having difficulties that he figured were drug-induced. Nobody—absolutely no one—warned him that you cannot go cold-turkey, that you have to taper off. So what happened is that going cold turkey caused a psychotic break. He attempted suicide and was taken to the psychiatric unit of a hospital—and there the presiding psychiatrist diagnosed him as having "schizoaffective disorder".

BB: Totally ignoring the fact that his was a common reaction to cold-turkeying.

JW: Precisely. And so he put John David on a number of additional drugs.

BB: So now your son was on a cocktail of different psychoactive drugs, all pulling his brain in different directions, right?

JW: Yes, and when he was released, my husband and I were given misinformation. We were told that our son had to be on drugs for the rest of his life and without them, he'd experience more psychotic episodes.

BB: What a frightening thing for parents to hear from a doctor! And did you at the time believe what you were being told?

JW: I was terrified! But it never crossed my mind to question it. And you know, people around me like my sister were very supportive of the status quo: The problem is that wherever I turned, I was getting misinformation.

BB: In fact, "garbage information".

JW: As I now know, but I had no clue back then. That was before I met you, Bonnie, because it was you who opened my eyes. And I believe that it was a happy coincidence that I ever encountered you....

BB: Again my apologies for taking you back there, Julie, and let me know if it's just too painful, but do you want to say something about how your son died?

JW: John David was suicidal—and let me be clear, it was because of the drugs he'd been taking. Now there was a gap of several years between the time when he had the first psychotic break and the time of his death. He was on and off the drugs. But the psychiatrist always wanted him *on the drugs*.

BB: And the reason John David kept going off was?

JW: He really didn't tolerate them well. Now he did have long stretches when he was fine. But then he'd remember what he called his "glory days" when he first started taking the stimulants—and I have since learned that's not atypical [stimulants, significantly, belong to the same category of drugs as "speed"]. And because at first it was fine—that's why you don't realize how deadly it can be. Anyway, back he kept going on the Dexedrine. Then the time came when he mostly went downhill. More and more he suffered. At one point, blatantly suicidal, he went to the hospital again, where he got no appreciable help. Then he left, came home, and not long thereafter jumped in front of a subway train. He ended the tragic suffering his own way. And what was left behind was a devastated family. It's been ten years now—and my husband and I have not gotten over it. We'll *never* get over it.

BB: Of course not. You lost your son. And though of course I'm talking figuratively here, in a way psychiatry *killed* your son.

JW: I believe that.

BB: Irrespective of their intentions, they made his life so miserable that he couldn't stand being alive.

JW: They did. They also fed him negative messages that were anti-hope. Like telling him that the best he can hope for now is maybe selling tickets in a box office, when he'd been a respected budding young theatre director.

BB: All the while, insisting that he had to be on these drugs for life?

JW: Precisely.

BB: So after his death, you started fighting back. You lodged a complaint with CPSO [The College of Physicians and Surgeons of Ontario]. And that was its own learning process. What did you find out about the accountability of psychiatry through availing yourself of the complaints process?

JW: That there *isn't* any accountability. That psychiatry is effectively left to police itself. The College bent over backward to retroactively change even the facts. They made it look like the problems my son was facing which they called "psychiatric" predated taking psychiatric drugs—when they didn't. As I saw them invent fact after fact, I was outraged. That they were okay with fabricating out of whole cloth a history that did not exist.

BB: And if I remember correctly, beyond that, you also found out that the system that you were up against was a circular in every way—you couldn't cross examine witnesses. And the people judging your complaint were all psychiatrists—all people with a vested interest in protecting the status quo.

JW: And it's not just a question of he-said, she-said—who do we believe? It's a question of fact invention.

BB: Which brings us to your activist years. About a year after your son's death the Coalition Against Psychiatric Assault held a groundbreaking international conference on organizing against psychiatry [see https://coalitionagainstpsychiatricassault.wordpress.com/events/past-events/psychout-a-conference-for-organizing-resistance-against-psychiatry/]. And the press got wind of it. Whereupon the conference and its organizers—including me—were utterly panned in the two front pages of *The National Post*—a major Canadian newspaper [for this article, see https://www.pressreader.com/canada/national-post-latest-edition/20100508/289712724936891]. That's how you came across us activists—from coincidentally reading that article, right?

JW: Yes, the reporter who'd written the article said that this conference was attended by what he called "crackpots".

BB: So what was the tipoff that something important was happening here?

JW: In addition to his gratuitous insults, he described some parts of the conference. And as I read the article, I became intrigued for I'd started to become deeply suspicious of psychiatry. Now by this point, I'd read my son's hospital file—and I was very angry at what I was now seeing as the system's betrayal of him. I also felt devastated, because I could see that I myself had not protected my son, had not done what I should have done.

BB: Julie, if I may interject, it wasn't your fault because you didn't know. And you know, I think a huge number of parents end up in

13 "I SO LOVED MY SON THAT I HAD TO PROMISE HIM THAT I'D DO... 179

precisely that situation. On the doctor's advice, they encourage their children to stay on these drugs. And one of the reasons, I suspect, few parents' voices get heard in protest against the system is that to do so, they would have to first face the part which they unwittingly played in the tragedy that unfolded. So let me you ask a question that I see as pivotal if we are to enlist parents as a resource: How did you arrive at a point where you were able to say: "I made a mistake. Like so many others, I believed what I was told. Not that at some point, I didn't have suspicions—and how I wish I had acted on those suspicions earlier—but now I can at least do something." How did you get there? Because that turnabout you did and that self-honesty, that's incredible! Cause as far as I can see, most parents just dig themselves in deeper—including after their child kills themselves.

JW: And who's to blame them? For who can possibly face something like this?

BB: Indeed, there is no blame accruing to parents here. But the answer to the question of who can face it is, obviously, *you* could—because you did. But *how* did you come to face it?

JW: I so loved my son that I had to promise him that I would do everything that I could.

BB: Are we talking about when he was still alive?

JW: No. After John David died, I read his medical record and I could hear his voice in these files. What I could see is that he had not acted foolishly by trying to go off the drugs. It was clear that for the most part he had a very astute understanding of what was being done to him—and he wanted it to stop.

BB: And your activism ever since has to a degree been your own way of keeping faith with that voice that you found in John David's medical record?

JW: Yes.

BB: That's incredible! What a brave and wonderful thing that you pulled off here!

JW: Thanks, Bonnie.

BB. So with this history, you walked straight into the antipsychiatry activist group Coalition Against Psychiatric Assault—which likewise amazes me. You were a mother who began with almost no critique of psychiatry. You were an accountant and so minimally a fiscal conservative. And you walked into a veritable hotbed of left-twing activists. How did you feel about being in our midst?

JW:	I was so curious. And I'd been so devastated that I was forced into a position that I think we should all live in—of open-mindedness.
BB:	But we must have seemed very strange to you.
JW:	Perhaps, Bonnie. Nonetheless, what struck me right from day one is that you had a very clear position, that you were incredibly articulate. And you knew things that I needed to know. What I quickly realized is that however you seemed to Joe Brean [the reporter who wrote the *National Post* article], you were brilliant people who knew truths that I in particular needed to learn.
BB:	And you did. For the next few years you entered a truly steep learning curve.
JW:	Thanks to you. You urged me to read Thomas Szasz [foundational theorist] and books by all sorts of other scholars—and I did begin to be able to really deconstruct psychiatry.
BB:	You sure did. Now within short order, you yourself became a knowledgeable critic of the psychiatric drugs—someone who helps gather and disseminate accurate information. For instance, you and your husband supported the research team who came together to reanalyze study 329. Would you like to tell the readers about study 329?
JW:	Study 329 is one of the many examples that exist of sham research. And Dr. David Healey, who was one of the people who headed this research [for background information, see https://davidhealy.org/the-troubled-life-of-study-329-the-consequences-of-failure-to-retract/], was convinced that the randomized control process that permits drugs to be approved is a badly flawed and manipulated process, which it surely is. If people knew what really happens in these processes, they'd be horrified.
BB:	So this particular study that the team that you were on was reexamining is connected with the drug Paxil [an antidepressant], correct?
JW:	Yes.
BB:	And what the team that you supported did is acquire the original data from drug trials that had not previously been made available and re-analyze it? And the conclusions that they reached were more or less the opposite of what appeared in the original article on the study?
JW:	The conclusions they reached were the *total opposite*. Let me give you a bit of background. The manufacturer—GlaxoSmithKline—

13 "I SO LOVED MY SON THAT I HAD TO PROMISE HIM THAT I'D DO... 181

was in hot water when the New York attorney-general charged them with fraud with respect to their public statements about Paxil; and as part of a settlement, they agreed to make the data on Study 329 available.

BB: So now you could get your hands on the data?

JW: Only theoretically, Bonnie. You see, what GlaxoSmithKline [GSK] did is allow you as reader to see individual pdfs of key documents through a viewer—but you could not save or duplicate any part of any of them. So one of the researchers in the UK spent eight months viewing these files and one by one and copying down the information.

BB: So now you had in essence recreated the data. And you were ready to perform a reanalysis. Give me an example of some of the differences between what the original GSK-sponsored article had stated and what your re-examination of the data showed.

JW: The 2001 article said that the data showed that Paxil was a safe and effective treatment for adolescents with serious depression. And what our re-examination of the data revealed is that it is neither safe nor effective. And what we saw is that original data had been manipulated [for an article that goes into the difference as well as into background information in vivid detail, so the reader can judge for themselves, see https://study329.org/].

BB: Of course, it was. As is more or less standardly the case. And so exposing manipulated research in this way is one of the things that people can do as an act of resistance. More generally, they can also educate about the drugs. Now in the very process of being involved in reanalyzing study 329, you were educating. But you've also been educating about the drugs in other ways. You and your husband, I believe, are also now the principal people running the enormously valuable website on people's SSRI stories [to view this popular website, go to: https://ssristories.org/]. How about introducing the reader to that site?

JW: It's a website that was started in the early days of the web by Rosie Mysenburg and two of her friends. She did it because she'd had an appalling experience on Prozac. Anyway, from her own personal experience she was acutely aware of how utterly inaccurate the standard information given about these drugs are. And she swore that she would get real information out there.

BB: So she created this website called "SSRIstories.org". And after her death, you and your husband, at the instigation of Dr. David Healey, maintained and added to this website. And the site is filled with a plethora of horror stories of what actually has happened to people who take these drugs.

JW: Yes.

BB: Julie, let's back up a bit. For readers relatively new to this area, could you explain what SSRIs are?

JW: It is the current major class of antidepressants. It is the selective serotonin reuptake inhibitors [serotonin is a neurotransmitter that these drugs target; Prozac is the most well known of these antidepressants].

BB: So the psychiatric mythos is that depressed people are depressed because they have insufficient serotonin—this, in the total absence of any indicator that there is anything whatever wrong with their serotonin levels. Now in reality, yes, the drugs act so as to increase the recipient's serotonin level. The psychiatric hype is that this addresses the problem. The reality is, it impedes the proper functioning of the brain by forcing a build-up of serotonin. Whereupon the brain fights back; then you have what is called "die-back"; and in the end you have a brain at war with itself, correct?

JW: Yes, and you've described that brilliantly in your book [Chapter 7 of Burstow 2015]. But to put it simply, when you start "messing with body chemicals" you create no end of problems.

BB: You surely do. Now the website you're overseeing is a constantly growing resource. It now contains over six thousand stories.

JW: More even than that.

BB: And these are stories that have made the newspapers—they are that famous?

JW: Yes.

BB: So: You have all these stories about people who have been damaged by the SSRIs, how it happened and how their lives played out?

JW: In addition, I'm coding the stories, so you can search by categories. For example, I now have a category containing hundreds of stories of people being killed by the police after an incident of mania that was clearly drug-induced. Also categories of suicide where the original story of course as it appeared said, that *despite* taking antidepressants, the person killed himself.

13 "I SO LOVED MY SON THAT I HAD TO PROMISE HIM THAT I'D DO... 183

BB: Whereas what you could make visible is that it is rather *because* the person took antidepressants, they killed themselves?

JW: Precisely. In doing work of this sort, you see, you learn to read these stories with a "new eye".

BB: So one of the utterly invaluable things you are doing is teaching people how to "read with a new eye", if I may put it this way. And that has been and continues to be a major part of your activism— teaching people how to read, how to deconstruct, while providing them with very accurate information.

JW: That's exactly what I'm doing. I make real information available, thereby making it possible for people to read their own experiences differently, in essence, to see through the misinformation they've been fed.

BB: Which is a sizeable contribution. That said, as valuable as such work is, the rub is that for decades, we've had a huge amount of accurate information out there, whether on the web, in books, or in printed journals, but that has not substantially changed the public awareness or for that matter altered the use of these drugs. So what else do you think we need to do to turn the situation around?

JW: That for sure is "*the question*". My own sense? I think we need to win more law suits.

BB: So launching law suits should be a major strategy?

JW: They're *one* avenue. I certainly wouldn't want to pin all our hopes on that avenue. However, I know that it can have an effect. A complicating problem with this route, though, is that the pharmaceutical companies have been able to control the bad publicity that would ensue if they lost their case by making a practice of settling out of court any suit that they suspect they'll lose. They thereby additionally ensure that precedents that could cause them trouble down the road seldom get on the record.

BB: All of which limits their value. Nonetheless, they surely are valuable. In the end, the pharmaceutical companies' overriding interest is profit—and this can affect the bottom line. What other promising avenues do you see?

JW: We all try to reach out through social media. Through talking to students. Then there's the invaluable work that people like you and Simon do [Simon Adam, an assistant professor of nursing at York University] By incorporating critiques of psychiatry into your courses, you are influencing the next generation of thinkers. And yes, I think it has an effect. That said, as you pointed out earlier, knowledgeable people have been drawing attention to inconsistencies and have been educating for decades—so why isn't the message getting through to the general public? You know, I think about that all the time. And my sense is it's attributable to the massive money that the psychopharmaceutical industry pours into misinformation, advertising, and cooptation.

BB: That is surely a humungous part of what we are up against. Were it not for the massive amount of money the pharmaceutical companies invest in propaganda campaigns and in downright cooptation of the research process, we'd have won this fight eons ago, for we've proven our points a thousand times over. Then adding to this problem is the enormous credibility given the medical profession, as Robert Whitaker points out, including and especially by the media [see Chap. 4]. So another question: How do we re-awaken the investigative instinct of the media? Something important at the best of times but which is critical now that we are facing an undeniable crisis.

JW: And what you're referring to here is?

BB: Over the last 5 years, the psychiatric/psychopharmaceutical assault on children has been growing exponentially. What's been happening? The Murphy bill was passed in the US—and what this legislation mandates is that once children are of school age, every single one of them will have to be diagnosed by a psychiatrist. This is an unparalleled invasion of children and of families—and if other jurisdictions started passing similar legislation, it could alter in a massive way what it means to be a human-being-in-this-world [for a more detailed discussion of this, see Chap. 5]. We are similarly looking at astronomical numbers of children being diagnosed with ADHD [Attention Deficit Hyperactivity Disorder] and placed on stimulants—way more than at the time your son John David was on them. Moreover, there are now initiatives afoot to have ADHD drugs declared "essential medicines" by the World Health Organization—drugs, note, overwhelmingly prescribed to children [see Chap. 14]. And if that initiative is successful, it will multiply by a good twenty times over the amount of these drugs most every country around the world has to have on hand. In short, we are looking at an unprecedented assault on children. And here is where people like you come in. Let me suggest that our best line of attack for combating this is precisely mobilizing parents, which in essence, brings us back to the focus with which we began.

JW: I surely do see your point.

BB: So how do we go from the situation that we have today, where parents largely follow doctors' orders and go along with the medication of their children—or worse still, join organizations that actively promote the medical model—to one where parents take in what is happening and transform themselves into an antipsychiatry force in their own right? My own personal hope is to see change happen here on two levels: One is where parents begin to seriously question what is happening and begin accessing or creating very different resources for their children. And two, where they band together and become a political force in the world. Now you are one of the people who did this kind of turn-around as a parent. So you are the expert here. So Julie, I am asking you, how do we facilitate such a shift? Or to put this another way: How do we help parents arrive at the different level of consciousness so that they can turn themselves into a formidable force in this fight?

JW: I think we have to get to the educators. I know that in Toronto, the school boards push the teachers to buy into and to promote the medical model.

BB: They surely do. Though I should note in passing, it goes way beyond the beliefs of teachers and members of schoolboards. They are *textually obliged* to be the eyes and ears of psychiatry via a hierarchy of documents that in Ontario, for instance, can be traced right up to governmental boss texts [an institutional ethnography term; see Burstow 2016]. Schools in that sense have very much become an intrinsic part of the psychiatric regime of ruling. That said, yes, we have to reach the teachers and school administrators. By the same token, we have to reach the press, because if the stories they told were different, parents would surely respond differently. For similar reasons, we have to reach the doctors. But what that leaves out is directly going to the parents themselves, that is, approaching parents as if they were or could be a formidable force in their own right. The point is: Parents, if united, can stand up to school boards. Parents, if united, can stand up to the psychiatric establishment. Parents can collectively stand up to the state. And please note, were such a force unleashed, it would be unstoppable. For parents concerned over the welfare of their children are more credible to the average person than school boards, than professionals, than the state itself.

JW: But you know, parents take their cue from teachers.

BB: They surely do, and they also take their cue from doctors. But the answer cannot be, first we have to change what teachers say, then we have to change what school boards say, and then we have to change what doctors say. We absolutely have to use those routes, but we can ill afford to just depend on those routes. Moreover, it is far too "derivative". The voices of parents should be their *own voices*, voices that arise out of *their own experience*, not primarily out of what they are told by others. So how do we help parents create *their own* counter-narrative?

JW: You know, there's a problem with the way children are now raised. When I was young, while we were told to respect adults and to respect authorities, a strong emphasis was nonetheless placed on questioning, on critical thinking, on thinking for yourself. Now people just go with "consensus". They have stopped thinking for themselves.

BB: And of course, we need to work on that. But our awareness of that larger problem cannot just be another way of putting off directly reaching parents. This is an incredibly powerful untapped resource. Think of it: If hundreds of parents started screaming, "You are destroying our children. With the blessing of the state which is supposed to protect us, here's what this institution has done to my son, my daughter, my baby—the story of abuse and of failure to protect would be all over the media and before you know it, the general public would be up in arms.

JW: You know, I've met a number of parents who are well aware that something is terribly wrong. Many have their own websites. They talk together on the phone.

BB: All of which is terrific. But my sense anyway is that it needs to expand. And we need something beyond parents talking to one another on the phone and creating websites.

JW: You are suggesting, are you, that parents need to come together and organize?

BB: Correct. How can we help the parents of psychiatrized children arrive at a position where they can turn themselves into a militant force in world? You know, one of the things that we could do just to spark off such a mobilization is a conference precisely on the psychiatrization of children—one that is first and foremost aimed at parents and to the extent possible, run by parents. We could also incorporate parents' voices into more broadly focused social movement organizations—something which we've already begun to do—though so far I've not seen this handled well.

JW: This, I'm relatively unaware of. What have you seen, Bonnie?

BB: Well, for example, there is a small but vital US group called "Draining Psychiatry of Respect". And it brings together statements by radical and at the same time highly credible "mental health experts" like David Cohen [a professor of Social Welfare at University of California] and me with statements by parents who have lost their children to these drugs. But too few parents are involved, and at least one of the parents involved has as yet little idea of how to be an activist. For example, her statement lacks emotional power. Additionally, shortly after a shooting in a bar in the US., she was on the internet saying that it is not the availability of guns that were the problem but the psychiatric drugs that the shooter was on. Whereupon, she publicly joined the National Rifle Association [NRA]. Now there is no question but that the drugs were the major problem, but joining the NRA in tantamount to "shooting yourself in the foot". So not only do we need to be prepared to help parents begin to organize themselves, we need to help them to actually master the ABC's of political organizing. On what is and what is not good strategy. Likewise, we need to help them arrive at an understanding of the science. I am thinking that teach-ins could help with all of this.

JW: We'd need people to turn up with an open mind. You know, in the early days, had I come across writings like yours, I wouldn't even have stopped to open the book.

BB: The difference was the personal experience, right?

JW: It was the personal experience, Bonnie. So the question is: How do we get to people before it's too late? How can we get to people steeped in the so-called conventional wisdom before utter tragedy sets in?

BB: Off the top of my head?: By reaching out to people when they are just beginning to have doubts. This is a time where there are niggling questions at the back of their mind, even if they are mostly dismissing them—and if we can help them look at the anomalies, they can build on that. And then we also need to reach out to people, where, as you put it, it is already too late, but they still don't want their child's death to mean nothing. Where they want to keep faith with their deceased child just like you have wanted to keep faith with John David. And this second group could potentially be of enormous help to the first. Who better?

JW: Well, I do have a group in the US that I can call upon at any time.

BB: So a query: How would you feel about CAPA and several members of your network either brainstorming together or creating a conference precisely on this question? Would that be something you would see as worth your time?

JW: *Of course* it's worth my time. And without question, I would be willing to invest my energy into this. But you know, we'd be up against a "PR monster".

BB: Absolutely. At the same time, besides automatically being credible to the general public, parents whose kids have been damaged by the drugs and who have been able to let themselves know that something awful has happened are already in a very different place than the average member of society. While they may not yet know the science, they know at a gut level that they've been tragically misled. And they have a clear reason to want to do something about it.

JW: I know from my own personal experience that that's true. So count me in. I am willing to do whatever it takes.

BB: Lauren Tenney [see Chap. 5] is also willing, though you bring something essential to the table that neither Lauren nor I conceivably could—the voice of a fellow parent. And in the work that lies ahead, you may well be one of the most important leaders that our movement has. For you have the lived experience of the parent. Anyway, see how the direction that's been emerging sits with you. That said, Julie, thanks for all the work that you've been doing. And thanks for this conversation.

JW: And Bonnie, thank you.

References

Burstow, B. (2015). *Psychiatry and the business of madness: An ethical and epistemological accounting*. New York: Palgrave Macmillan.

Burstow, B. (2016). *Psychiatry interrogated: An institutional ethnography anthology*. New York: Palgrave Macmillan.

A Relevant Publication by Julie Wood

Wood, J. (2015). Pilots crashing on antidepressants: A (not so) brief history. *Mad in America*. Downloaded August 29, 2018 from https://www.madinamerica.com/2015/03/pilots-antidepressants/

Julie's Added Comment

As parents, all of us have things we would like to go back and do differently. For most of us those things are minor, such as missed opportunities—and so there are ways to later go back and compensate for them. Not so for me.

I lost a person I loved more than anything in the world in part because I trusted him—he had always been responsible and shown good judgment—but what is of far more significance, I lost him because I trusted the medical system. There are many wonderful aspects to our medical system. Our family and several other people who I know have benefited greatly from it. Psychiatry is not among the positives.

When I think about what people need to thrive and prosper emotionally—and these are things like safety, personal space, autonomy, respect, intimacy, the chance to contribute, and the opportunity to be heard—I marvel at how easily we have been duped by psychiatry. The point is that what psychiatry either directly involves or leads to is the antithesis of all these good things: Here is a profession that pretends it can improve our well-being by isolating us, labelling us disordered, reducing our confidence, nullifying our opportunities, and drugging us. The drugs numb our emotions, dull our cognition, and stop us from giving "a damn about anything". They likewise induce sudden rages, make us miserably restless, and take years off our lives. Psychiatrists, moreover, act as if they can intimately know 50 or so people at any given time simply by talking with them in an artificial environment for 45 minutes each week. They claim that in this manner, they know more about what we need than we do. *And we buy this?*

Strange though this may seem to you, psychiatry is about creating problems, not solving them. We need to observe more critically what is really going on. When psychiatry gets hold of you and you have a bad reaction to the medications that they give you, all the side effects will be attributed to inherent disorders. You run the very high risk of having your life destroyed in what will ultimately be an agonizing, demoralizing process. It's bad enough when we accept this for ourselves. We should never allow our precious children to fall into this trap.

Insofar as you are able to stop it, do not let anybody, in the name of mental health or however else they describe it, suck into the psychiatric system your son, your granddaughter, your neighbour's kid, or your godchild. Be vigilant and take in this horrible truth—that the people enter the psychiatric system do NOT get better, they get worse. It is not "in spite of" all the help they receive that psychiatrized children have greater and greater problems as they age. It is rather because of it.

If you want me to elucidate further or you just want someone to interact with over all this, please feel free to contact me at SSRIstories.org. I can tell you about the hundreds of kids who hang themselves every year, the dozens who are shot by police, the many many more whose lives are derailed, all because of psychiatric drugs. And I just might be able to answer some of the questions that you have.

CHAPTER 14

Epistemicide: Dialogue with "Global Mental Health" Critic China Mills

China Mills is a faculty member in Public Health at City University of London in the UK. She is likewise an author, a member of the editorial collective of Asylum Magazine *(for a discussion on this magazine, see interview with Ian Parker), a researcher with a strong focus on "mental health" developments in India, a disability theorist, a discourse analyst, an ally of the survivors'/users' movements, and finally, and most especially, a leading critic of the Movement for Global Mental Health, and moreover one with a powerful anti-colonial frame. I first met China a few years ago when, like Ian Parker, she agreed to write a chapter for an earlier book of mine. And to my good fortune, our paths have continued to cross.*

BB: China, as a researcher, you're known for such related areas as the critique of the Movement for Global Mental Health; Fanon scholarship [Algerian anticolonial psychiatrist; see Fanon 1952/1967], psychiatry as a colonial enterprise, and critical discourse analysis. For the benefit of readers not versed in these areas, would you like to begin with some clarifying remarks? A tall order, I agree.

CM: (laughing). Oh wow, Bonnie!

BB: (laughing). I know. I've just asked you to explain the world, haven't I?

CM: Okay, I'll have a "go". Let me just say that it's common for people in the global north not to know what the global mental health

© The Author(s) 2019
B. Burstow, *The Revolt Against Psychiatry*,
https://doi.org/10.1007/978-3-030-23331-0_14

191

movement is, though not people from the south. Which I find interesting (laughter). It is a movement, I would argue, that originated largely from psychiatrists in the global north, and it stands for the scaling up globally of "mental health services" which generally means "medications" and other forms of what people call "psycho-social support" to people in lower income countries specifically, though also globally. And they tend to embed their case in a human rights framework, which largely boils down to the right to access "treatment"—which is interesting, because the people who oppose the Movement for Global Mental Health also mobilize human rights, but in a very different oppositional kind of way. Which is both confusing and interesting. Technically, the movement dates back just prior to 2007 and the publication of influential articles in the *Lancet* [leading U.K. medical journal], but the actual idea and practice of globalizing psychiatry dates back way earlier. And it's a very similar logic.

BB: And this historical piece is fundamental to understanding what we are facing now. The point is that the penetration of psychiatry into non-European countries didn't simply begin a handful of years ago but is part and parcel of the centuries-long invasion and colonization of other countries.

CM: Absolutely. And this history is totally left out of the accounts of Global Mental Health enthusiasts.

BB: Which is terrifying, because such is the essence of what is happening here.

CM: I keep grappling with is what is new about this movement while trying to historicize it, placing it in a much longer history—and, without question that history is colonial.

BB: And Fanon was clear that the problems for which people in the "colonies" were being given psychiatric diagnoses stem directly from colonialism. That people were being diagnosed and treated for what were normal responses to colonialism.

CM: Absolutely, and that's why his work is so important. Because he was a psychiatrist who saw very clearly the colonial underpinning and he talks about how psychiatry and the psy disciples [a concept originating with Foucault which refers to psychiatry, psychology, social work. and related disciplines] reconfigures resistance to colonialism as mental illness and how this reconfiguring is used to both "treat" people and delegitimize the resistance.

14 EPISTEMICIDE: DIALOGUE WITH "GLOBAL MENTAL HEALTH" CRITIC...   193

BB: Yes. So you're one of the leaders who critique this area. And that critique strikes me especially crucial at this time when the psychiatric complex is on the hunt for ever new markets, which right now, is largely being secured through the Movement for Global Mental Health, along with allies like the World Health Organization, the World Bank, and the International Monetary Fund. It's undeniable that the quest for markets is a primary motivator. And whatever else the Movement for Global Mental Health brings, psychiatry is front and center. Correspondingly, we know from history that seemingly sincere attempts to modify biological psychiatry by adding elements of social support such as the Movement for Global Mental Health unquestionably does, yields little more than psychiatry with add-ons. Biological psychiatry continues to dominate.

CM: Yes.

BB: Now China, you raise an excellent question in your book [Mills 2014]. Having articulated the enormity of the problems caused by psychiatry in the west, you ask: If this doesn't work, why export it? However, you *don't answer* the question, almost as if there were no clear answer. But let me suggest there is one and it is obvious. It gets exported because exporting it is in the interests of psychiatry and the psychopharmaceutical industry and because in the final analysis, colonizing and expanding markets is what the movement is all about. In your otherwise terrific book, it's as if you are reserving hope that global mental health can somehow be "cleaned up" and become benign. Which parallels what psychiatric reformers have been claiming since the seventeenth century. I don't believe it can be "cleaned up". I'm putting you on the spot, I realize, but do you believe that there can be a "good" global mental health movement? To put this another way, have you been pulling your punches or do you believe that this cleaning-up job can be done?

CM: That links to something that I would change were I to rewrite my book (laughter).

BB: Interesting. What would you do differently?

CM: It relates exactly to what you just said. The very title of my book "Decolonizing Global Mental Health" is problematic. I shouldn't have called it that for I don't think that it's possible to decolonize Global Mental Health.

BB: I'm relieved—also touched—to hear you say that.

CM: (laughing) My students and I, we often discuss questions like: Is it possible to decolonize practices like Global Mental Health or psychiatry, and would there be anything left if you tried? You know, even to assume that you can decolonize is to treat those processes as much more separate than they are. Psychiatry and psychology are bound up with colonial thinking and scientific racism.

BB: Yes, it is at the center of the philosophy. Practitioners can want to be antiracist, but how can they be when they don't understand the racism inherent in saying that some people's bodies are inferior and we need to alter those bodies?

CM: Yes. And I don't even have a language to talk about it because they are so tightly interwoven with one another.

BB: Agreed, and when you think about it, China, even the idea that the solution to the problems faced by people from completely different cultures lies in the belief systems and practices of the very others who create a good part of their problems in the first place is incredible. How could anyone believe that? It is a bizarre belief at best.

CM: (laughing). It is, yes. Now whether or not that makes me "anti" some of these practices, I don't know. But I don't think that it's possible to decolonize them. And as you put it, neither do I think that it's possible to "clean them up".

BB: You know, when countries in the global south join with psychiatric forces in the global north, I feel like I do and like Roland Chrisjohn does [see Chap. 2] when we see Indigenous people forming alliances with psychiatrists. Part of me wants to scream out: Stop. They are going to try to decimate your culture. Of course the psychiatric colonizers give people reason to believe that they will tone down the psychiatric aspects and they start bringing in Indigenous practices like healing circles but the point is, despite this seemingly benign coming together of different cultures, psychiatry is a ruling regime whose ultimate agenda is to control and expand.

CM: And we see that in the way that drugs and psychiatry are used in "humanitarian" efforts. The giving comes with a price. Now some groups know very well that those psychiatric packages come with such problems. And accepting those frameworks is strategic for them; it's a way to get funding. In India, I have seen that happen.

BB: I can surely appreciate that. And *of course*, it is a way to get resources—and indeed resources that are often desperately needed. The problem is that the "gift" comes at the cost of their culture, not to mention the health of their population. I truly get that it can initially look like a good tradeoff, or, as you put it, a strategically sound course of action but many have discovered to their chagrin that it's far too big a price to pay.

CM: Absolutely.

BB: And this seeming charity is itself both part of and a type of colonization.

CM: Yes. In India, where I've done a lot of research, you can see that the biopsychiatry and pharmaceutical approach to mental health dominates. You know, I have spent many years talking to different nongovernmental organizations and different people, including user and survivor groups in India who would very much like to promote a non or at least "not only" pharmaceutical approach, but they struggle to get recognition.

BB: Additionally, the second you say "not only", let me suggest you've lost the battle. Because the best you can end up with is biological psychiatry with add-ons. And that's basically what we have everywhere. That's the problem, not the solution. And of course, if you don't have money, or power, or recognition, these compromises look reasonable. But let me ask you something. What if Gandhi said, "It's way too extreme our seeking liberation from English rule. Let's just have an England-India alliance in which we have a little bit of one and a little bit of the other?"

CM: (laughs). I get your point. And in a way that speaks to my uncertainty about whether or not to be antipsychiatry. You see, I am not sure if I am "anti". Nonetheless, never once have I seen a space where psychiatric understanding coexists equally with other approaches. As you've said, if they are present, they nearly always dominate.

BB: However nicely they may play in the beginning, in the end, they *always* dominate. We can trace this dynamic through centuries. The whole reason that psychiatry turned to drugs *is* to dominate. The beauty of saying drugs were needed is that it helped them drive out other therapists, other competitors for dominance in the madness turf.

CM: You know, I have been trying to focus on what we might call psychiatric thinking rather than speaking of psychiatrists versus non-psychiatrists, because in India, there are heated debates between psychiatrists, and just to simplify this, there are whole groups of psychiatrists who want to keep the power to diagnose and to treat solely in the hands of psychiatrists. And then there is a whole other set of psychiatrists—some of them influential players in the Movement for Global Mental Health—who want to see a diffusion of what I'm calling psychiatric thinking. And you see this play out in Global Mental Health where people talk about task-sharing. They want to share some of the power and skills of psychiatrists with community health workers. And it's fascinating how this has been incorporated into different technology. So smart phones have "apps" that allow you to identify and supposedly manage different kinds of mental health problems, with community mental health workers using those apps to diagnose. And also in global north countries, though increasingly also in low and middle income countries, you see the *Diagnostic and Statistical Manual* simplified even further. It is written into technology, and community health workers are using that.

BB: So everyone can be a reductionist, can be a psychiatric oppressor. Isn't that what we are seeing here? That everyone can be a psychiatrist?

CM: (laughing) Yeah.

BB: I am reminded here that in the 80s a social work colleague of mine sent me an article he'd just written making the case that social workers should be allowed to prescribe psychiatric drugs. I was a social work professor at the time, which is why he was sending it to me. So what do you think?, he asked. Of course, I couldn't support this direction. Why ever would we want *more professionals* authorized to do the very thing that is harming people?

CM: And this position taken by the "progressive psychiatrists" concerns me for the very reasons you're concerned. But in Global Mental Health, psychiatrists who take that position are seen as radical. And to add to this, in India you also see people involved in local spiritual practices working alongside psychiatry, and psychiatrists will go to the temples or the spaces where those forms of healing happen and distribute medication there, working alongside those healers. Meanwhile, the underlying model of psychiatry never gets challenged.

14 EPISTEMICIDE: DIALOGUE WITH "GLOBAL MENTAL HEALTH" CRITIC... 197

BB: Precisely. And what a worrisome development! To shift the focus slightly, the last person I interviewed was Peter Breggin, and it has brought me back to a conundrum that I've known about for years—that those of us on the left are at least as big a problem in this area as the right is. The left tends to believe that as long as we are socializing everything and so everyone has access to psychiatry, we are doing the right thing.

CM: Yes, and in England, the talk is all about fighting to keep services that we already know are highly problematic.

BB: We are "snowed" by the concept of services. We immediately think something horrible is happening if there is a cutback to services for we are predisposed to think of anything called "services" as worthwhile. And psychiatry really isn't a service. It's a disservice. Now it is showered with so much funding that a little bit of real service ends up bestowed on people who come into contact with it—such as people having someone to talk with or a place to stay for the night—but that is hardly the essence of psychiatry.

CM: Absolutely and psychiatry or a psychiatric way of thinking is so tightly entangled with what everyone would agree constitutes services—services, as you say, such as dealing with homelessness—that it is difficult to separate it.

BB: And in North America anyway, we now face a horrid development called "linked services". So people are told, yes, we'll provide housing for you, but only if you first agree to take psychiatric drugs. And I imagine you have a version of that in England.

CM: We actually see welfare payments made conditional on either going to therapy or taking medication. So the linking is with psychotherapeutics as well. Indeed with all of the psy disciplines.

BB: Incredible! And there are two problems with the rest of the psy disciplines. One, they are colonized by psychiatry. And the second is that regardless, they are a colonizing force in their own right.

CM: Absolutely. They do the same work, the same kind of reconfiguring. So while it is critical to talk about psychiatry specifically, it is vital to keep in mind that there is an underlying logic that they all share.

BB: Yes. The individualizing, the decontextualizing, the pathologizing, the emphasis on conformity.

CM: I totally agree. And even when professionals resist psychiatry, they simply pathologize from within their own discipline. How to explain? ... Well, a good example of this is in a school in a disadvantaged area that I've interacted with. The teachers were quite resistant to medicalizing children's behavior or distress. Nonetheless, that resistance was inextricably linked with a psychologizing stance. So teachers would say things like: Well, we don't think it is a "brain disorder" but it is obviously an "attachment disorder".

BB: Which is a psychoanalytic way of handling it, and while psychoanalysis isn't brain-damaging, it is likewise pathologizing and depoliticizing.

CM: Yes.

BB: As you have brought up children, let's move on to the control of children. I don't know the statistics in the UK or India. But I do know that ADHD is one of fastest growing diagnoses globally and that the attack on children is astronomical.

CM: The US has led the way here. And the globalization of that particular diagnosis, literally, you can almost watch it happen in real time.

BB: So in your research, you yourself are seeing it pop up in country after country?

CM: Absolutely, especially among the middle class, but then it slowly shifts to the working class. Now research shows the growing use of that diagnosis in middle income countries. But it is starting to go to the others. You know, every couple of years the World Health Organization publishes what it calls "Essential Medicines". And psychotropic drugs are included. Three or four kinds of antipsychotics, three or four kinds of antidepressants, etc. And you can actually see in the minutes of meetings of the World Health Organization where they discuss what should be on the list, that there is a lobby to try to get ADHD drugs included as essential medicines. And to be clear, being on the list means that absolutely every country should have a supply of those drugs. So I am watching to see what happens in regard to that lobby. But these discussions suggest that we will likely see ADHD drugs massively increase globally. Also what is significant here, a lot of countries have shifted from using the WHO's ICD [International Classification of Diseases] to using the DSM [Diagnostic and Statistical Manual of Mental Disorders—a product of the American Psychiatric Association].

14 EPISTEMICIDE: DIALOGUE WITH "GLOBAL MENTAL HEALTH" CRITIC... 199

BB: Good to know. They are both horrible but the DSM is more in the pockets of the drug companies.

CM: Yes and the DSM criteria for ADHD is much looser. So it is easier to get an ADHD diagnosis.

BB: As with all its other diagnoses.

CM: Indeed. It's worrisome that these even exist. It's likewise worrisome they are the only schemas and these are used to diagnose everyone in the world. And there is even a discussion of the two manuals merging.

BB: To a degree, it's already happening. For years now, they've worked at making the two manuals compatible with each other.

CM: Yes!

BB: And this is empire building.

CM: A very good way of describing it.

BB: A few hundred years from now, historians will talk about this as the Psy Empire because what has transpired has all the markings of empire. A global ruling that continues to spread, that is dominated by one philosophy and accompanying agents of enforcement.

CM: It's amazing.

BB: That said, I wanted to turn to similarities and to one difference between the two of us linguistically. Even when not referring to the global, we both employ the word "colonization" to talk about psychiatry. The reason in both our cases, I suspect, is that psychiatry strongly resembles colonialism in how it works—and so it is a deep metaphor. And so I talk about psychiatry's colonization not only of the world generally but also of the disciplines surrounding psychiatry. You do this too, but you also apply it to another situation, which application strikes me as inaccurate—though I'd like your current thoughts on this. You refer to the drug companies' colonization of psychiatry. And I'll tell you why I think that's inaccurate: When you colonize, you invade. Psychiatry got *saved* by the drug companies. They weren't *invaded* by them. With the spread of psychoanalysis, which clearly wasn't medical, and with the rise of nonmedical therapies and therapists, psychiatry was on its last legs [for a detailed discussion of this, see Burstow 2015]. It got saved by the claim that emotional problems are medical, that people need to be drugged—which makes it the province of doctors. That does not sound to me like psychiatry was colonized. That sounds to me like an unholy alliance was struck between psy-

200 B. BURSTOW

chiatry and the drug companies, leading to expansion of psychiatric drug use that is in both industries' interests, though I surely do get that individual psychiatrists may *feel* as if they've been colonized.

CM: Hmm … I think what you're saying is true. I seem to have fallen here into the words used by various psychiatrists who claim that the profession has been colonized by the drug companies. So, yes, I agree, it's a misuse of the word. That said, to go to the larger issue, I am aware that there are debates about whether or not critics should be calling what psychiatry does colonizing.

BB: Sure and the question here is whether or not we are falling into racism. And it's an extremely important question. Here's my take on it: My sense is that because psychiatry was an integral part of what everyone agrees is colonialism and because it is inherently racist and operates like colonialism, it is at very least a deep metaphor and as such, a metaphor we should be using. And we are missing out psychiatry's historical place in colonialism and the inherently racist and subjugating nature of the discipline and its operation when we fail to use it. You know, my own take as a member of this movement is that it is problematic when we sacrifice analyses just because we are afraid of making comparisons.

CM: Yes, it closes down thought, doesn't it?

BB: Here's how I see it: If you are using a word simply because it makes what has happened to you look more serious, that is appropriation and is totally problematic. On the other hand, if a word that you are adopting refers to a process that parallels in important ways what you have undergone, and if in addition the oppression being discussed is inextricably tied to that other oppression historically, then it's a *deep* metaphor.

CM: I like what you are saying here. And I think that psychiatry and traditional coloniality are so tightly bound to one another that there is, as you say, a depth to the metaphor.

BB: This reminds me, besides that some Mad in America authors told their readers that they cannot use the term psychiatric slavery and I think that's misguided for the metaphor is deep, moreover, because slavery is a generic term, not one owned by only one enslaved people, on top of that, readers were likewise told that they it was unacceptable, indeed was antisemitic, to compare other oppressions to the Holocaust. Now to zero in on the Holocaust claim per se, "Holocaust" is a very particular term meaning "place of the burning" and it was specifically invented to cover what transpired in Nazi Germany and so care is needed here; and just using the name as it's often been used to refer to other people's and even other species' oppressions can be problematic. Nonetheless, saying this is different than saying that comparisons with the Holocaust should not be made. As a Jew who was born during the Holocaust and who is an expert in both antisemitism generally and the Holocaust in particular, I don't find it inherently antisemitic. Making comparisons is a valid thing to do in general—and what a shame that we are closing down knowledge creation! And more particularly, when psychiatric survivors in particular use a Holocaust metaphor, how could it be appropriation? Besides that an important comparison that can be made between what happened to Jews and what happens to psychiatric survivors, the Holocaust is a vital part of psychiatric survivor history. It is important to remember that hundreds of thousands of "psychiatric patients" were systematically murdered by the Nazis, and this paved the way to the systematic annihilation of the Jews. Bottom line: Comparisons are vital to analysis; we have to proceed carefully and knowledgably of course; but it is a bad mistake just to rule them out by fiat.

CM: Absolutely.

BB: Okay, more general topic: A lot of us who have been in this fight since the 70s or 80s would like to see some development or other that actually puts psychiatry on the ropes; and we haven't come close to seeing it. What we've seen instead is the continued expansion of psychiatry. Now we've for sure seen an enormous growth of good critique, but this has not substantially impeded psychiatry. Rather psychiatry continues to grow by leaps and bounds. What would be a strategy for reversing this? And I realize that's a tough question but it is a critical one for otherwise, social change won't happen.

CM: And I absolutely agree. There's been so many incredibly deep critiques of psychiatry—both from psychiatrists and others—one has to ask: how many more are needed? Or are we finding out that this strategy isn't the way to go?

BB: Obviously we have to create these critiques and exposés. Nonetheless, we surely need to come to grips with the fact that what we are doing is woefully insufficient. And a comparison may help highlight why. To stick with India, what if instead of going on strike and openly defying English law by marching to the sea to mine salt, Gandhi did nothing more that pen critiques of England's colonization of India? India would still be under English rule. Obviously when it comes to oppression, more than critique is needed. Now I would welcome other views on this but as far as I can see, there are two ways to go, and one is direct opposition. This is what Gandhi did when he said: We'll break your laws and we'll obstruct business as usual. And the other is that to create experiments, trying out new ways of helping people—now I know that adherents of the Movement for Global Mental Health believe they are doing the second; but they are not—they are spreading/ imposing psychiatry with minor modifications.

CM: Agreed. Postcolonial critique is informative here. They talk about how one of the most powerful things about colonialism in India— and I'm sure this applies more broadly—is that colonialism frames both the arguments for it and the arguments against it. So even when you are trying to be anti-colonial, you are using colonial frames.

BB: An excellent point. Which is why you have to get behind these, rise above them, throw them out. They can't be a starting place. You know, I'm an anarchist, not a centrist, a believer in small self-governing communities. And I see the local and its protection, together with its practices and vocabulary as critical. The local is after all where the lifeblood of people is. It is the culture. It is the society. It is the grounding.

CM: Yes.

BB: That said, to get back to the more general point, I would like to see the movements challenging psychiatry become a lot more activist. The big question that people keep asking seems to be: How can we get government to cooperate with us?—and I think the question is misguided. What we should mainly be asking is: How can we apply pressure so strategically that we win the battle?

CM: Indeed. And to go back to what I said about colonialism framing the dissent to it, how much is psychiatry also doing that? How much is psychiatry framing the "anti" as well as the "pro"? How much is it coopting the very critique of psychiatry?

BB: A salient question, and I would suspect that the answer is "enormously", for indeed, psychiatric concepts operate in the vast majority of the critiques. Critics use the word "mental health", for example. They use the word "diagnosis". They use almost the entire psychiatric framework. How can you do that and think that you have a critique?

CM: And to add another dimension, looking at local practices and discourses that happen not only in the UK but also in the global south can be informative for they may do the job of psychiatric critique without explicitly being framed that way.

BB: Absolutely. For among other things, they are reclaiming culture. And instead of focusing on psychiatry in a tunnel vision kind of way, we need to devote more energy toward addressing the vital question: How can we help others bring back local practices which have been at least partially obliterated by psychiatry?

CM: Yes. And there are some brilliant examples of that in India. Now to be clear, some local practices are as awful, violent, and disempowering as psychiatry. Also the plurality we are still seeing may disappear if psychiatry globalizes further. Nonetheless, there is still a pluralism of understandings in India of why someone might be distressed.

BB: Which is excellent.

CM: At least there is a choice. And there are ways of different perspectives co-existing that are very interesting. So how do we preserve and engage with that sort of thing, that sort of pluralism?

BB: I totally believe in such pluralism—just to be clear, though, I just don't think psychiatry has a place in it, albeit medicine more generally does. But do we need pluralism? Of course, we do. That's what got driven out with the spread of psychiatry.

CM: Absolutely. And to pick up the thread of colonization, you can see the almost exact same language within much of the writings on Global Mental Health that you see in classical colonial writings. You see the same elbowing out or demonization of other forms of healing because they are seen as irrational. And you can see that in the slogans.

BB: Yes, in the use of concepts like "rational" and "progressive" and "moving beyond superstition", even in frequent repetition of phrases like "evidence-based research".

CM: Yeah. And you know, there have been incredibly important movements and critiques against psychiatry, but generally the underlying logic remains the same.

BB: Agreed. And the appeal to the government tends to worsen the problem.

CM: And that's what makes what's happening in many of the low and middle income countries interesting because often the government isn't involved. Many of the programs in India I work with get nothing from the government. And in many ways, they are disadvantaged for they have no resources, but at times that is the beginning of something very good and very different. All these alternatives.

BB: Which is what we need. Government needs to stop the push toward professionals and/or we need to operate outside of government. The very idea that the well-being of people is something that should be in the hands of professionals is nonsense. And if you don't tie yourself to official funding, you are less likely to go in that direction, whereupon diversity enters in.

CM: You know, there's a Portuguese theorist called De Sousa Santos who works in Brazil who talks about "epistemicide" [see De Sousa Santos 2014]. Operating as if there's only one way of thinking about things is engaging in what he calls epistemicide.

BB: In feminist circles in North America, we have a similar concept. We talk about epistemological violence—where the mainstream or hegemonic way of thinking violently drives out every other way.

CM: Yeah, and that's an interesting concept which different movements, diverse though they may be, could unite around—being against epistemicide in whatever forms it takes, whether psychiatric or general neoliberalism.

BB: I totally agree. And I would add that these kinds of critiques are very big in feminist courses. And while we are touching on feminism, I did want very quickly to bring up an issue that likewise alarms me. It is how the feminist critiques of psychiatry which were once so central to our movement have almost disappeared. How do you think that's come about? Or are you hanging out in difference venues and seeing something different?

CM: You may be happy to learn that there's a strong feminist critique of psychiatry in India.

BB: Great to hear—and yes, I'm delighted. And from your work, do you think that's because women in India are very much grappling on a larger level with the problems presented by the patriarchy?

CM: (laughing) Yes. Also many writers explicitly frame their critique of psychiatry that way because the framing of madness is so explicitly gendered in India. But when it comes to North America, yeah, I know what you mean.

BB: And this is a major problem, for psychiatry is very clearly a product of the patriarchy. We still have the phenomenon, for instance, of two to three times as many women as men being subjected to electroshock. There is no way around the profound sexism underlying such statistics. And there are similar problems with respect to racism.

CM: And the disappearance of gender and race theorizing very much pertains to the user and the survivor movement. We see resistance to thinking about sexism, white privilege, or white supremacy within survivor spaces.

BB: In all cases, yes, we surely do.

CM: And I agree with you that established feminist and anti-racist critiques tend to get lost in the newer spaces.

BB: And we can ill afford for them to get lost. When we look at current problems, current practices, we need to be clear what ruling(s) they're a part of.

CM: And there's a tendency to think of everything as new. And yes, we need to see the new, but we can't lose sight of established critiques.

BB: For doing so means losing historical understanding and inevitably losing depth.

CM: Absolutely.

BB: Which is as good a place as any for us to end. This has been a very interesting conversation, China. Such an important area—and yes, I agree that it is extremely telling that so many people in the global north know virtually nothing about the movement to globalize psychiatry—when we, after all, are the crux of the problem. And what a gift to have heard from a sophisticated thinker so deeply involved in the global south!

CM: It's been such a pleasure, Bonnie.

BB: China, thank you so much for this interview.

CM: No, Bonnie, thank *you*. It's always lovely to have an excuse to talk to you.

206   B. BURSTOW

References

Burstow, B. (2015). *Psychiatry and the business of madness*. New York: Palgrave.

De Sousa Santos, B. (2014). *Epistemologies of the south: Justice against epistemicide*. London: Routledge.

Fanon, F. (1952/1967). *Black skins, white masks* (L. Markmann, Trans.). New York: Grove Press.

Mills, C. (2014). *Decolonizing global mental health: The psychiatrization of the majority world*. London: Routledge.

Representative Publications of China Mills

Howell, A., Mills, C., & Ruston, S. (2017). The (Mis)appropriation of HIV/AIDS strategies in global mental health: Toward a more nuanced approach. *Globalization and Health, 13*(44), 1–9.

Klein, E., & Mills, C. (2017). Psy-expertise, therapeutic culture and the politics of the personal in development. *Third World Quarterly, 38*(9), 190–208.

Miller, L., & Mills, C. (in press). The politics of global mental health governance. In R. Moodley & E. Lee (Eds.). *Routledge international handbook of race, ethnicity, and culture in mental health*. London: Routledge.

Mills, C. (2017a). The mad are like savages and the savages are mad: Psychopolitics and the coloniality of the psy. In D. Cohen (Ed.), *Routledge handbook of critical mental health* (pp. 205–212). London/New York: Routledge.

Mills, C. (2017b). Psychopharmaceuticals as 'essential medicines': Local negotiations of global access to psychotherapeutic medicines in India. In J. Davies (Ed.), *The sedated society: The causes and harms of our psychiatric drug epidemic* (pp. 227–248). London/New York: Springer.

Mills, C. (2017c). Dead people don't claim: A psychopolitical autopsy of UK austerity suicides. *Critical Social Policy, 38*(2), 302–322.

Mills, C. (2018). 'Invisible problem' to global priority: The inclusion of mental health in the Sustainable Development Goals (SDG). *Development and Change, 49*(3), 843–866.

Mills, C., & Davar, B. (2016). A *local* critique of global mental health. In S. Grech & K. Soldatic (Eds.), *Disability and the global south: The critical handbook* (pp. 437–452). New York: Springer.

Mills, C., & Hilberg, E. (2018). The construction of mental health as a technological problem in India. *Critical Public Health*. https://doi.org/10.1080/09581596.2018.1508823.

Mills, C., & LeFrançois, B. (2018). Child as metaphor: Colonialism, Psygovernance, and epistemicide. *World Futures, 74*(7–8), 503–524.

China's Added Comment

I loved reading through our discussion, Bonnie, while simultaneously experiencing that jarring feeling of having one's words captured and written down. Throughout our conversation, I keep catching glimpses of something that we mention and then move on—a niggling, like a wobbly tooth, around the question of being antipsychiatry. I still don't know what I think about this, although I greatly valued the chance to talk through these issues with you.

In my own thinking, I've tried to stop centering psychiatry all the time and, instead, think about the wider logics of the psy disciplines more broadly and their linkages with practices of categorization and classification, decontextualization and individualization, and the ways hierarchies and moral economies are formed through these processes. While I do think psychiatry does specific things and we shouldn't lose sight of these, I think it is important to keep in mind the shared practices across all things 'psy'. But, also, to be alert to worldviews and practices that are not psy-centered, and so act as alternatives but not as critiques that revolve around psychiatry. I worry that by being 'anti' psychiatry, we risk psychiatric logic shaping our resistance.

I mentioned to you my regrets about naming my book "Decolonizing Global Mental Health"—yet another niggle. This regret comes because since publishing the book, I have had the chance to speak with, as well as read the work of, some awesome thinkers who live, experience, breathe, and/or study colonialism, de-colonialism, postcolonialism, and anti-colonialism. From these folks, I see much more clearly now the trap (some would say impossibility) of trying to de-colonize colonial systems and structures. Mental health categorization and classificatory politics are examples of these systems—inseparable from the wider background of violence, hierarchization, and coloniality that is often defined as normal, necessary, and rational within modern, and many postcolonial, nation-states. For me this highlights *the pervasive interlocking of classificatory politics, of which mental health categorization plays a central part, and coloniality, meaning that tweaks in the name of social justice in one part of the system will often leave the wider system in-tact*

CHAPTER 15

"The Movement Is an Intrinsic Part of Who I Am": Dialogue with Bonnie Burstow

In what is a turn-about, this—the last of the interview chapters—is with me, Bonnie Burstow, as interviewee. As the reader is already aware, I am an academic, a leading antipsychiatry activist and theorist, a philosopher, and a radical feminist therapist. The person interviewing me is Oriel Varga. Oriel is an activist in the area and someone with a law degree who has been called to the bar (at present, she is working on her doctorate and is not practicing law). I have known Oriel for a decade, with the relationship between us being a combination of mentor/mentee, fellow activists, fellow artists, and friends. How fortunate that as a student of mine, Oriel was able to make visible that how and what I teach is in its own right a way of being an activist!

OV: Okay, Bonnie, to plunge straight into this, you've been involved in the antipsychiatry movement for ions. Just what got you started?

BB: Well, like lots of people, my initial involvement stemmed from seeing vulnerable folks around me psychiatrized. My father, who was subjected to over a hundred ECT "treatments", also several high school chums, who had fallen upon rough times. What I saw was the harm done to them by people in power who didn't appear in the least to understand the travails of being human, and my heart ached for them. Fast forward a few decades. In the 1970s, I took a job with an organization that worked out of Queen St. Mental

© The Author(s) 2019
B. Burstow, *The Revolt Against Psychiatry*,
https://doi.org/10.1007/978-3-030-23331-0_15

209

210   B. BURSTOW

Health Centre [a huge Toronto psychiatric "hospital"]. Now to be clear, we weren't working *for* the institution—we were an independent community organization trying to get people *out of* the institution. And here I witnessed ever more horror shows. Now several years after I left this job, to my surprise, a psychiatric nurse employed there who's always appreciated my radical perspective, called me up. "Bonnie," she said, "they just killed another 'patient." What happened is an inmate had died and she had lifted the file, hoping that there was something I could do. "Bonnie," she went on, "they subjected Aldo to such a problematic combination of "meds" that it killed him; they shipped him to Toronto Western where he was declared 'dead on arrival'. You're political and I suspect have connections. Anything you can do here?" Sweating profusely—I was that nervous—and playing a Deep Throat sort of role [Deep Throat was the secret informant involved in Watergate], upon receiving a copy of the file, I proceeded to spirit it off to people in the New Democrat Party of Canada [local socialist party]. Within days, the issue was raised in the provincial legislature, and the media were all over the story, henceforth known as the Aldo Alviani Affair [see http://www.psychiatricsurvivorarchives.com/phoenix/phoenix_rising_v1_n3.pdf.].

OV: So that was the Alviani Affair?

BB: Yup. You know, I was myself a student at the time. And some good for sure came of the action, with the inquest that ensued resulting in some degree of change—though, in all honesty, not much. Now I also knew that while this action had been successful, it wasn't exactly the way forward as an activist. Several years later as a radical feminist therapist who was an outspoken critic of psychiatry, I took the next step, started writing articles for Canada's antipsychiatry survivor magazine.

OV: *Phoenix Rising?*

BB: Precisely. And before I knew it, I was a member of the collective and to an appreciable degree, had cast my lot in with survivors. And once there, I never looked back.

OV: I sure do see how this happened. And what's kept you active all these years?

BB: In part the obvious lies told by psychiatry and the horror of what they do to people but also the terrible double binds in which this population finds themselves. The fact that their perfectly reasonable objections to being shorn of their rights and bodily invaded are automatically invalidated, even taken as sure-fire proof that they need to kept under "control". I might also add, on a level nothing short of existential, this community had become *my people*, this liberation movement an intrinsic part of who I was. What goes along with this, what was happening to these people served as a window onto what was wrong with the world generally and by contrast, in the movement against it, I saw glimpses of the type of society that we needed to build.

OV: I sure do get that. I sense that being a woman also figured in.

BB: Indeed. Most of us women know deep down that psychiatry is a vehicle of the patriarchy.

OV: I know that your early work—a high percentage of your scholarly articles, for example—was steeped in feminism.

BB: Yes, as were the hordes of workshops I provided for social service workers. At the time, additionally, I was regularly used as a consultant by feminist counselling agencies. Places like Women's Counselling Education and Referral Centre [a Toronto agency] were eager to avail themselves of my radical feminist/antipsychiatry approach for this was one of the moments of feminist awakening.

OV: Do you still incorporate feminism?

BB: Absolutely. For example, besides my teaching and nonfiction, my latest novel—*The Other Mrs. Smith*—is an intrinsically feminist novel. How it could be otherwise when these oppressions intersect so?

OV: While we are on the issue of intersectional oppression, how do you bring critical race analysis into your antipsychiatry praxis?

BB: In part, by calling attention to the blatantly worse treatment that people of color receive at the hands of the institution. For example, by highlighting the hugely disproportion number of Black folk who are saddled with the one diagnosis that virtually gives the authorities carte blanche to intrude—schizophrenia—then inquiring ideologically, historically, materially into how this comes about. I should add, just like we have an insufficient emphasis on gender in our movement—and at this point, alas we have—we positively "suck" when it comes to race—problems we direly need to address.

OV: Something I'd like to see also. To turn to a very different issue, about 15 years ago, you and Don Weitz started a vibrant and long lasting antipsychiatry organization called "Coalition Against

212   B. BURSTOW

Psychiatric Assault" [CAPA; see https://coalitionagainstpsychiatricassault.wordpress.com/] and it is still going strong. To what do you attribute its exceptional longevity?

BB: Curiously, what's made the largest difference is not what people think. We have a damned good analysis, but that's not the primary reason we've lasted so long. Here's what social movement literature tells us: Ninety-five percent of small social movement organizations fold within 5 years of starting. And what light does research shed on why that small percent last longer? It has little to do with ideology—though we'd like to believe otherwise—and successes naturally help, as do attending to the needs of your members, as does being "cutting edge" but it's not the central factor—prosaic though this is, it comes down to materiality. Those that last longer primarily do so because they can access resources—and that is surely the case with CAPA. What have we by way of resources? A steady stream of interested and interesting students from my courses. A free room to meet in. Space for holding major events. Technical assistance. And so my advice to groups just starting up, naturally, put your focus on principled praxis but don't ignore the material.

OV: Interesting and obviously consonant with Marxist analysis. To zero in further on your activism per se, your creation of an antipsychiatry scholarship aside—and we'll get to that later—what do you regard as the most successful action that you've been involved in, and to what do you attribute its effectiveness?

BB: Well, if we can go back to the 1980s—it's Ontario Coalition to Stop Electroshock's three-day sit-in in protest of ECT in the Minister of Health's Office. We received a huge amount of press as a result, the vast majority of it very positive, and the public began getting highly interested in the issue. And why was it so effective? Because having taken training on how to pull off civil disobedience, as survivors and allies, we handled the situation skillfully and the public took note and were impressed. What likewise helped us, no one had ever done anything similar before. And here's the takeaway lessons for activists: Strategize and train—don't just "wing it". And what is new, what takes them by surprise—has a far stronger chance of working than the so-called "tried and true".

OV: Yes, that's something that I've always appreciated about you. More than anyone else in the movement, you've always emphasized

15 "THE MOVEMENT IS AN INTRINSIC PART OF WHO I AM"... 213

strategic activism. So, Bonnie, in general, as you see it, what does good strategy look like?

BB: Gandhi's campaigns are the paradigm. What is good strategy? Good strategy involves having a campaign where one event follows another. And the ideal strategy involves catching the opponent on the "horns of a dilemma", such that however they respond, they lose. A good example of this is Gandhi's historic march to the sea to mine salt in direct violation of the British prohibition against local inhabitants mining salt. So Gandhi and his followers were visibly breaking the law. Which left the British oppressor with only two options: They could ignore the "the violation", in which case Gandhi wins for he has shown he can successfully defy the might of the British empire. Or they can arrest and maybe attack Gandhi and his peaceful followers for doing nothing but mining their own salt in their own country. In which case, Gandhi also wins, for he makes manifest to the world the injustice and the brutality of the British Empire. So there in a nutshell is strategic activism at its best. You have to get your oppressors in a position such that no matter what they do, they lose.

OV: Interesting.

BB: Now the next thing, as I've said, is you don't engage in an isolated act. You need to build an orchestrated campaign. Now in all activism where you are using non-violent resistance—and that's what we're talking about here—you have to apply pressure so as to get the oppressor to effect change; and for that you need leverage.

OV: Which comes from where?

BB: Gandhi's leverage arose from the sheer numbers involved—you can hardly jail the entire population of India. And in most struggles, one can go on strike and jeopardize the economy—also leverage. Here's the difficulty: Psychiatrized people have almost no leverage. And that problem is not going to disappear overnight. What adds to it, this is a group that gets drugged and has difficulty sustaining action.

OV: So what's the answer?

BB: Would that there were "an answer"! You use whatever leverage you can find in the situation confronting you.

OH: Yeah, I've noticed us doing that. That said, have you ever seen any group in the movement pull off a really good piece of strategic direct action?

BB: Actually, I saw an exceptional beginning of one. Remember the 2003 MindFreedom Hunger Strike?

OV: Say more.

BB: This was an impressive and highly intricate hunger strike organized by MindFreedom [for details, see http://www.mindfreedom.org/kb/act/2003/mf-hunger-strike/fast-for-freedom]. Its purpose? To force the APA [American Psychiatric Institution] to acknowledge that they had no credible evidence that what they called "mental illness" was intrinsically biological or that psychiatric drugs were beneficial. So they put hunger strikers at the center of the action, from which of course, they garnered the press, and they brought in highly credible professionals like Breggin to assess whatever evidence APA brought forward. Nothing short of brilliant. Now indeed the APA responded with their "evidence". Whereupon the panel of experts handily demonstrated the invalidity of that evidence. So far so good. But there the campaign stopped. Now Michael Weinberg—the mastermind behind the action—was well aware that there had to be follow-through but no one went with him—and here's the rub: If you cannot sustain and build a campaign, you fall seriously short of successful strategic activism. And alas, what we have here is a population with limited energy and a limited number of people who can continue to turn up. And one consequence of this is, like with traditional prisoners—psychiatric inmates are in dire need of the prolonged work of allies. Now allies were centrally involved in the MindFreedom hunger strike. But that was still not enough.

OV: I see.

BB: The point is, minimally, with such actions, you are in for a one, two-year campaign.

OV: So long-term work?

BB: Precisely.

OV: Important to know. So let me ask you, Bonnie, how do you compare the strategy of the antipsychiatry movement to that of the mad movement?

BB: These are perspectives and sub-movements—not strategies—and I don't see either of them as committed to any particular strategy. And it is precisely because of the void here that as an antipsychiatry activist, I came to create the attrition model of psychiatry abolition.

15 "THE MOVEMENT IS AN INTRINSIC PART OF WHO I AM"... 215

I in essence created a meta-model that can be turned to for long term strategizing by antipsychiatry activists.

OV: Could you give us an overview of the model?

BB: The attrition model of psychiatry abolition is predicated on the awareness that you can't get rid of psychiatry over night. If you want psychiatry abolition, you have to wear away at the institution bit by bit. So it's a metamodel to keep activists from straying away from the long-term goal. It pivots around the use of three key questions, to be turned to when assessing or planning possible actions. To paraphrase, they are: One—if successful, will the action being contemplated advance the long-term goal of psychiatry abolition? The second question is: Does it avoid adding legitimacy to the current system? The point is, otherwise—oops—you're going in the wrong direction. And the third question is: Does it avoid the pitfall of widening psychiatry's net? What's the third question mean? If you can think of these institutions as huge nets that catch people up in their rule, the more people they can entangle in their net, the more damage they can do, and so you never want to participate in an action whose probable consequence is widening that net, irrespective of however otherwise good it might seem.

OV: So the model is essentially something groups can use to keep themselves on track.

BB: Precisely. And CAPA has often used it to come to consensus over actions over which members are seriously divided.

OV: Fascinating!

BB: It helped us to decide to actively support an action in the US aimed at banning the use of ECT on children. How so? Banning an injurious treatment for one part of the population is demonstrably moving in the right direction. To cite an example of a harder decision it helped us make, folk in the mad movement wanted us to support an institutionally supported walking tour of the walls at Queen St. Mental Health Centre, historically built through the forced labor of "patients". And the question divided us, with some feeling that since psychiatry looked bad, there was no problem giving our support, while others were uneasy. Not having consensus, we turned to the attrition model. What going through the questions showed us is despite how bad the psychiatry of the past appears, the action makes current psychiatry look good by comparison for they are cooperating with this tour, and as such,

216 B. BURSTOW

> if we joined this action, we'd be lending legitimacy to the current system. The upshot, we opted not to participate [for further details on his model and the use made of it, see Burstow 2014].

OV: So, Bonnie, what's the worst mistake you ever made as an activist?

BB: Well, it was a mistake that *all of us* made together. And it goes back to the heyday of Ontario Coalition to Stop Electroshock. You'll find more about this in my dialogue with Don Weitz [see Chap. 8], but in short, the Coalition's efforts to date had been monumentally successful. We had the active ear of press. We had the public onside. We had the local boards of health and the province actively considering what to do. Then we made a colossal blunder. We asked for an official investigation into electroshock. They gave us what we asked for, which is all they had to do to kill the issue. Over the years during which the official investigation took place, the momentum against shock that we had so carefully built up evaporated. And when the report finally did come out, besides being deficient, it was never acted upon. The lesson here is never ask for an investigation. Rather, demand immediate action. Now the tragedy for us in Ontario is never again were we able get the vital question of ECT back on the public agenda.

OV: An important lesson here that it behooves us to remember.

BB: It is. Because if you ask for the wrong thing, you kill your movement.

OV: I can see that. I'd like to shift the conversation more at this point to you as an academic. Now while you've been an enormously influential and successful academic, you've also encountered obstacles, as people engaged in radical praxis often do. Could you give us a sense of those obstacles and how you, well, "speak back" against them?

BB: Sure. Now to be fair, I've not only faced obstacles I've also received a lot of support, for which I am truly grateful. But have I encountered obstacles? Yeah, everything from direct interference—an example being an overt threat that the credentializing body in social work would withdraw credentialization from the university who'd just offered me a position if they went ahead with hiring me—to things subtle but utterly systemic, such as lack of access to funding—for the big research funders do not fund research that problematizes psychiatry—something students in the area likewise

15 "THE MOVEMENT IS AN INTRINSIC PART OF WHO I AM"... 217

face. What adds to the problem is that you are treated differently at the university if you don't bring in money. More generally, there have been attempts—albeit only sporadically—to interfere with my courses, also to interfere with conferences that I was mounting.

OV: How about giving us an example of concrete interference, together with how you dealt with it? This is the kind of thing that those of us who are students need to understand.

BB: Here's one: When I was teaching in the Social Work program at The Winnipeg Education Centre at University of Manitoba, one day the head of the program brought me a letter he'd just received from the Department of Psychiatry saying that in the interest of my students having a balanced view of psychiatry when right now they were only getting mine, psychiatrists should be allowed to come into a course I was teaching and to inform my students of their perspective. The irony of the situation was that psychiatry was barely touched on in this course. Anyway, unsure what to do, the head of the program handed me the letter and asked me to respond. No greater gift could have been given to me for I was able to figure out instantly how to respond. Remember my earlier point about catching the opposition on the horns of a dilemma? That's exactly what I did here. I wrote back saying, "Thank you very much for your concern over my students having access to only my perspective. And in the interest of my students receiving a 'balanced view', I have no problem with psychiatric faculty coming into my course and explaining their position—but *if and only if* in the interest of your students *likewise* acquiring a "balanced view", I similarly am invited into your courses." Here's why he was caught on the horns of a dilemma: Since I was a better researcher and better presenter than anyone in psychiatry, if he agrees to the blatantly even-handed offer that I was making, he loses. And if he says no, he is tacitly acknowledging he has something to fear here, in which case, he also loses. It goes without saying that we never heard from either him or his colleagues again.

OV: What an awesome story!

BB: I similarly turned the tables when several faculty at University of Toronto objected to the PsychOut Conference that I was instrumental in organizing [a 2010 international conference on organizing against psychiatry] And students were elated upon my making public my reasoned and principled response to the objections raised, whereupon much to the chagrin of the naysayers, they began flocking to the conference in droves.

OV: My take is, your default mode is to use "push-back" as "teachable moments".

BB: An insightful observation, that—and yes!

OV: Brilliant. Now Bonnie, you recently were promoted to full professor. And your students, colleagues, and fellow activists came together to celebrate. And people talked very personally of how central you've been to their lives and to their research. Do you have any advice for graduate students who want to follow in your footsteps?

BB: Never just follow in anyone's footsteps. Figure out what your own center and passion is. Become the very best researcher, the very best thinker that you can possibly be. Never tone down what you have to say. And approach objections to what you are doing as an opportunity to educate.

OV: Which brings us to the question of the endowed scholarships. But a year or so ago, you created the world's first antipsychiatry scholarship [The Bonnie Burstow Scholarship in Antipsychiatry]. And I have to say, this generous gift of yours is going to go a long way to helping students wanting to take up antipsychiatry research. Now I have noted from a recent blog article or yours just how difficult and challenging the fight was to gain university acceptance for the scholarship [see Burstow 2018]. Could you share a few tips on how to handle this for people who might want to endow similar scholarships?

BB: Let me begin by saying that to pull this off you need to be 100% principled—you can't make anything up—you also have to be 100% visionary, and you have to be 100% practical. Rally your supporters and allies, and one by one, deal with every objection cast in your path. And never forget that you can leverage strategically the value of academic freedom. Moreover, you need to stand your ground. The one thing that you cannot do is compromise.

OV: But what about the power of the multinational pharmaceuticals to stop you? What about the vested interests within academia?

BB: A very real problem that you need to strategize around. My response to every threat, incidentally, was to "increase the emphasis" on academic freedom. Now is academia coopted? You betchya.

That said, Oriel. as I see it, "academia" is not just this "thing" out there. *You* are academia. *I* am academia. And we as actors can do something of significance in how "academia" is created and recreated. That said, just to slip this in, I hardly see either scholarship endowment or academia more generally as the major arena where the fight for justice is occurring or will occur. It is simply one of the avenues available to us.

OV: Got it. And what do you see happening if others endow similar scholarships around the world?

BB: While for one thing, we would have changed the discourse. And we'd have a growing area of research—for the scholarships will attract students. Moreover, this area would have been given ever more legitimacy by the sheer existence of the scholarships. We'd also have changed the material reality. We'd have in essence put concrete money into the pockets of students intent on pursuing research in the area who otherwise might not be able to. Now I said we are creating new discourse, which is true, but what's happening goes beyond even that. We're at the same time facilitating what Foucault (1980) calls "the insurrection of subjected knowledge"—in this case, the knowledge of the mad.

OV: We surely are.

BB: And we are helping it perk up through academia, which in turn, bestows legitimacy on it. So we're both creating new discourse and further legitimating discourse that has been disallowed and inferiorized throughout the ages.

OV: And in line with standpoint theory, it's important to focus on the perspective of mad people in the face of the centralizing of the "sane" perspective, just like it's been important to focus on the perspective of women given the centrality afforded the perspective of men.

BB: Absolutely.

OV: And by doing so, we're decreasing the power of psychiatric hegemony. Is that part of what you had in mind when creating this scholarship?

BB: Truthfully, it's part of what I *always* have in mind. And funding scholarships is just one of the many ways that I myself interrupt psychiatric hegemony. I likewise aim to interrupt it in the various projects that I've created, in the books and articles that I've authored, in the radical actions of which I am a part, in the very courses that I teach.

220   B. BURSTOW

OV: Which brings us to your trauma course. I had the enormous privilege of being your student in that truly incredible course where we approach trauma in a way that "speaks back" to psychiatry. And in this course, you had us do something very difficult for us as students. Which is to stay entirely away from psychiatrizing perspectives on trauma. So staying away from labels, and approaching the crises that people face in living as political and philosophical issues. I personally found the course enormously powerful. Could you tell us a bit about your trauma perspective approach to problems in living?

BB: Just to clarify for the reader, it's not just a trauma perspective—note, psychiatry too has a trauma perspective. It is explicitly a *counterhegemonic* trauma perspective.

OV: And the context are historical and current oppressions. And your perspective is a way of countering psychiatry's truth claims.

BB: Yes, truth claims are countered. But what it does far more is expose psychiatry in a different way. What psychiatry does is strip traumatized and other people in difficulty of their contexts. Stripped of context, they often look "crazy" because what you have reduced them to is a grab bag of "symptoms". And now you can categorize them hegemonically and so on. So the course begins from the premise that we shouldn't be looking at context-less symptoms. We should be looking at the whole person, which necessarily includes their context. Well, the second you bring back context, people no longer look crazy. They merely look like fellow human beings struggling like we all do with the problems that beset them in their lives. And the contexts we need to factor in are not only the immediate context, but also what happened to them earlier, what *is* happening to their community now, and what has happened to their community historically. So we need to look at them in their totality, and in the process, look at the injury and oppression involved and find ways of both validating them and helping them navigate a far-from-ideal world. At which point, of course, the DSM looks utterly irrelevant. Other critical aspects of the course and perspective are using an inclusive definition of "trauma practitioner"—one hardly limited to counsellors or even professionals—the emphasis placed on transferring one's skills to the community, and learning how to bridge the literal/metaphoric

15 "THE MOVEMENT IS AN INTRINSIC PART OF WHO I AM"... 221

divide when interacting with people who live in "alternate realities" [for details, see last chapter of Burstow 2015].

OV: And what advice have you for counsellors or therapists, or what you call "befrienders" so they don't psychiatrize?

BB: A good place to begin is: a) identifying and b) throwing out the terminology. If you use the terminology, as we know from institutional ethnography, one way or another, you become "institutionally captured" by it. So it means cleaning up your language and looking at the very real injury that happens to people—at an individual level, a community level, in the here-and-now, historically, and systemically. It means more generally being prepared to validate rather than invalidate, to help people resist and counter oppression as needed, and to advocate. It means knowing scientifically as well as spiritually the harm done by psychiatry and seeing as an intrinsic part of your job helping your clients protect themselves from that. Moreover, it means maintaining a vision of a better world and allowing your sense of that to guide you.

OV: To focus in on survivors themselves, what advice have you for people stuck in the psychiatric system? What specifically interests me here is that there are people who get stuck in the system who don't want to take the "medication", don't see themselves as "mentally ill" and yet according to various critics, we have created our legal regimes such that the more people in this situation resist—and on some personal level, these resistors are antipsychiatry—the more likely they are to be pronounced "incapable" of making "treatment decisions". So how do they navigate their lives in the face of such contradictions and double-binds?

BB: Oriel, you've hit the proverbial nail on the head here. You are almost totally hemmed in by contradictions and double binds when pronounced "incapable". And in their actual resistance—which seems totally impossible—yes, herein lay antipsychiatry. My advice: Join with inmates similarly situated. Join with allies. On a more immediate and pragmatic level—and that too is crucial—find a lawyer with a history of sniffing out institutional blunders that they use to their clients' advantage—like a form not submitted on time. Stay calm or your very understandable rage or upset will be used against you. More generally, whether you are rejecting "treatment" or not, whether or not you are physically in the institution, keep in mind how "mental health professionals" read the world. Here's the thing: As members of society, most of us are sufficiently "sane literate" to know what not to say if we don't want to get locked up in a psych institution. So most of us know, for example, you don't go up to a "mental health professional" and say, "I'm going to kill myself and here's how I'm going to do it."—because they are going to incarcerate you. One thing I've noticed about psych survivors is while many are singularly adept, a disproportionate number are lacking the sane literacy needed to protect themselves. This is where befrienders and allies can really help. One type of assistance befrienders can offer is helping the vulnerable people around them become more adept at reading who they can and cannot share what with. On a more systemic level, whatever our situation and wherever we are in the world, in line with the CRPD [see Chap. 12] we should all of us pressure our respective governments to repeal the Draconian legislation on which such horrific practices rest.

OV: To focus in once again on psychiatry per se, in your book [Burstow 2015], you in many ways demonstrate the invalidity of psychiatry. Has psychiatry responded to your critique? And if not, what do you make of their silence?

BB: Psychiatrists don't read what I have written—let's be clear. Nor do they respond in any obvious way. What they do with me, indeed, what they do with all foundational critics—and note, that there are legions of us—is ignore us and keep spreading their propaganda. Why? In part because as Whitaker puts it [see Chap. 4], they are taken in by their own rhetoric, so "common sense" has it become to them. In part, because the strategy has proven to be eminently successful. That said, have they not responded at all? Not exactly. Students of mine who are workers in the "system" have been covertly threatened. That is, they've been cautioned that if they continue with me as their supervisor, their career is in jeopardy. Which amounts to a tacit acknowledgment that there is a counter-discourse out-there that is powerful and that they have something to fear.

OV: You saying that we need to continue the critique?

BB: Absolutely.

OV: One more topic I want to touch on. Bonnie, on top of being a teacher and a writer of nonfiction, you're also a novelist. Your terrific novel *The Other Mrs. Smith* brings in the experiential

15 "THE MOVEMENT IS AN INTRINSIC PART OF WHO I AM"... 223

through the use of first-person narration. How did you come to write this novel and what's your hope for it?

BB: Why I wrote it to goes back to the loss of public interest in ECT that I spoke of earlier. Fiction has the potential to bring the issue of ECT back onto the public agenda. The point is the public is moved by fiction. So my hope is that if enough people read it, we can stir up the public outrage needed.

OV: I know it's moved me—and powerfully so. How I hope to see a movie made of it! And to ask one final question, for I'm an artist too—what can allies who are artists do to help in the overall movement? And how do they prevent themselves from getting coopted?

BB: We surely need artists, for artists are society's communicators and healers *par excellence*. A reality, incidentally, I also stress in the trauma course. What can artists do? Incorporate the horror that is psychiatry into your art. Keep reminding yourself whose side you're on. Talk to survivors. Do art *for*, *with* and *alongside* survivors. And bottom line: never enter the psychiatric institution with your art for that lends the institution credibility and makes the oppressor and place of confinement look like part of the community. More generally, use your art as only you can, to help people know, think, feel, intuit on a deeper level, to help them fathom and truly appreciate what might initially seem alien to them. And in so doing, join in this part of struggle to build a better world. But Oriel, you yourself use art this way. I'm particularly heartened by the time you spend with others creating art for political events, patiently putting in hour after hour even when only a couple turn up to co-create with you.

OV: To me it's always worth the effort for art moves people and builds community. Optimal is when artists work with the community, joining with the oppressed, joining with social justice activists.

BB: Ah yes, the two of us have greatly overlapping visions.

OV: And on that note, Bonnie, thank you so much for this interview. As an activist, what stands out most for me are your pointers on strategic activism. Not that that's all. You know, every time we have a conversation, I come away with new understanding and new tools.

BB: Which, to be clear, says at least as much about you as about me. And Oriel, thank *you* for this interview, and thanks for your work over the years.

REFERENCES

Burstow, B. (2014). The withering of psychiatry. In B. Burstow, B. LeFrançois, & S. Diamond (Eds.), *Psychiatry disrupted* (pp. 3–16). Montreal: McGill Queen's University Press.

Burstow, B. (2015). *Psychiatry and the business of madness.* New York: Palgrave.

Burstow, B. (2018). *Three scholarships: The revolution continues.* Downloaded July 27, 2018 from https://www.madinamerica.com/2018/05/three-antipsychiatry-scholarships/

Foucault, M. (1980). *Power knowledge* (C. Gordon, Trans.). New York: Pantheon.

REPRESENTATIVE PUBLICATIONS OF BONNIE BURSTOW

Burstow, B. (1992). *Radical feminist therapy: Working in the context of violence.* Newbury Park: Sage.

Burstow, B. (2003). Toward a radical understanding of trauma and trauma work. *Violence Against Women, 10*(11), 1293–1317.

Burstow, B. (2005). Feminist antipsychiatry praxis: Women and the movement(s). In W. Chan, D. Chunn, & R. Menzies (Eds.), *Women, madness, and the law: A feminist reader* (pp. 245–258). London: Glasshouse Press.

Burstow, B. (2013). A rose by any other name: Naming and the battle against psychiatry. In B. LeFrançois, R. Menzies, & G. Reaume (Eds.), *Mad matters: A critical reader in mad studies* (pp. 79–93). Toronto: Canadian Scholars Press.

Burstow, B. (2014). The withering of psychiatry. In B. Burstow, B. LeFrançois, & S. Diamond (Eds.), *Psychiatry disrupted* (pp. 3–16). Montreal: McGill Queen's University Press.

Burstow, B. (2015). *Psychiatry and the business of madness: An ethical and epistemological accounting.* New York: Palgrave Macmillan.

Burstow, B. (2016). *Psychiatry interrogated: An institutional ethnography anthology.* New York: Palgrave Macmillan.

Burstow, B. (2017). *The other Mrs. Smith.* Toronto: Inanna Publications.

Burstow, B. (2018a). *Teaching counterhegemonic trauma courses: A "kickass" way to be antipsychiatry.* Downloaded August 6 2018 from https://breggin.com/bonnie-burstow/

Burstow, B. (2018b). *Three scholarships: The revolution continues.* Downloaded July 27, 2018 from https://www.madinamerica.com/2018/05/three-antipsychiatry-scholarships/

Burstow, B. (2019). From bed-push to book activism: Anti/critical psychiatry activism. In U. Gordon & R. Kinna (Eds.), *Routledge handbook of radical politics* (pp. 82–96). London: Routledge.

Epilogue

All books must end, and that, of course, includes this one. Nonetheless, if the architect(s) of the project have done their job well, the dialogues, narratives, and images which they have introduced into the world never quite end. And with that thought in mind, my hope is that the conversations which figure in this book will continue, both between the original dialoguers themselves and between others—both inside and outside this project—who come upon these threads. Also, that the words and images, even the sense of what it means to be alive that asserts itself in this book will continue to reverberate.

I know that many of these continue to echo in my head, inviting, at once, both reflection and action. While there are literally hundreds of words and images that stand out for me, and while different ones are prominent on different days, to name just a few, there is activist Don Weitz's gutsy decision to identify as a psychiatric survivor/activist *after having been a psychologist*, also his call for more direct action (see Chap. 9); there is Tina Minkowitz's seemingly out-of-the-blue dream that she was a lawyer, together with her implicit invitation to become active in lobbying states to bring their practices into conformity with the CRPD (see Chap. 12); there is Peter Breggin's and Nick Walker's urging us all to love one another (see Chaps. 3 and 10); there is archivist and grieving mother Julie Wood's deeply personal and heart-breaking statement, "It's been ten years now—and my husband and I have not gotten over it. We'll *never* get over it"—a declaration which is surely a signal for us to act, as is the model that

© The Author(s) 2019

B. Burstow, *The Revolt Against Psychiatry*,
https://doi.org/10.1007/978-3-030-23331-0

226 EPILOGUE

she provides of an everyday person responding to tragedy by courageously placing one foot after another and, in the process, turning herself into an activist (see Chap. 13).

There's the sheer determination and vision evident in Tatiana Castillo's words, "We don't just want to *change* the 'mental health system'...we are out to change society" (see Chap. 8); there is China Mills' compelling argument that we need to recognize and weed out all instances of "epistemicide", irrespective of what form it takes (see Chap. 14); there is Lauren Tenney's haunting warning that if we allow things to continue in the current direction, "in two generations we are going to have an entire society that has no idea what it means not to have a psychiatric label" (see Chap. 5). Likewise, gripping are the various strategic errors highlighted, together with clarifications of where they lie (see Chaps. 5 and 15)—and how essential learning from such missteps is to good activism!

Additionally, there are various projects introduced that in themselves serve as exemplum—from blogsites, websites, and magazines (e.g., Chaps. 2, 3, 7, and 13), to supportive peer-centered houses (e.g., Chap. 6), to participatory research projects (e.g., Chap. 5). There are not only reports of current and past projects but the beginnings of new projects in the early stages of being hatched (e.g., see Chaps. 5, 11, and 13). There are lessons that may only become obvious when you read several of the stories—such as that survivors have a special knowledge that the rest of the population cannot have and so need to be front and center. And then there's the enormously important discussions of intersectional oppression, including and especially, Roland Chrisjohn's uncompromising depiction of the psychiatrization of Indigenous people as "a continuation of genocide" (see Chap. 2).

In fact, the last of these moved and motivated me so deeply that before I had even sent the manuscript of *The Revolt Against Psychiatry* off to a potential publisher, with the help of students, of Indigenous communities, and of others, I had already mounted a conference at Ontario Institute for Studies in Education of the University of Toronto (OISE/UT) called "The Psychiatrization of Indigenous People as a Continuation of Genocide", with none other than Roland himself as keynote speaker, and with the audience jointly brainstorming what to do about the situation. "Build it, and I will come", Roland had responded minutes after my contacting him about the possibility (personal communication). And within months, together, several of us had built, it and he, indeed, had come, as did literally hundreds of others. Hopefully, it is the harbinger of mobilizations to come.

Questions: Will the seeds of Indigenous resistance planted by Roland take root? Will the international organizing intended to counter the escalating assault on children actually come about? Will we be able to facilitate a mobilization of parents? Can we protect our children? Can we change the face of academia—whether through creating scholarships and counter-hegemonic courses or in the very way we approach teaching (see Chap. 15)? Can we resuscitate our grassroots practices, including and, in particular, those eroded by colonialization? Can we create more constructive interchanges between the mad movement, the antipsychiatry movement, the neurodiversity movement, and the disability rights movement (see Chaps. 10 and 12)? And finally, a pivotal question to which all of us keep returning: Will we ever be able to rein in Big Pharma? Or for that matter, the academic psychiatrists who prop up psychiatry (see in particular, Chaps. 2 and 3)? My guess is yes on all counts—but only if we double and triple our efforts, only if we are uncompromising in our analyses and our actions, only if we avail ourselves of all the avenues open to us, only, as Tenney puts it, if we keep "reinventing ourselves" (see Chap. 5), only if we become increasingly strategic (see Chap. 15), only if we find ways to pull together. As such, this is an invitation to, at once, reflect more deeply, to network, and as Don Weitz puts it (see Chap. 9), "to up the ante".

In the same vein, but more generally, I would invite the reader to ask themselves: Which of the statements and which of these dialoguers most speak to you? Which are you avoiding? What are you being called upon to rethink? In what direction do they point? If you could imagine yourself taking a step in that direction, what would that step look like? And if there are unresolved issues in your life that prevent you from taking that step, how might you begin picking away at them?

There are additional questions that I am, likewise, inviting the reader to grapple with. Most but not all of these relate to issues on which there are significant divisions—I suspect, inevitable ones—between the different voices in this book. The biggest of the divisions, as China Mills' final comment highlights (see Chap. 14), is on the perennial question of abolition versus reform. So: Where do you yourself stand on this issue and why? And if, as is the case with several of the people who participated in these dialogues, you are "on the fence", can you imagine not being on the fence? To be clear, I am not suggesting that being "on the fence" is inherently or inevitably a bad thing, but it is critical to have a way of determining when it makes sense and when it does not. What concretely does that mean?—you may be wondering. To introduce a distinction that may be of service here, it is one

228 EPILOGUE

thing to be on the fence when you are uncertain about the validity of psychiatric claims. On the other hand, if your own analysis shows them to be utterly faulty, being "on the fence" can never just be a default mode. So the question to consider is: If you yourself see psychiatry's primary claims as foundationless, and if, in addition, you see their approaches as primarily and overwhelmingly harmful, what, if anything, would you take as an indicator that it is time to "get off the fence"? And in practical terms, how does "being on the fence" work? For example, how do you see resolving the conflicts that inevitably arise when actions that look good in themselves, nonetheless, seriously undermine abolitionist goals? To approach this issue from a slightly different angle, if you let yourself think in terms of the *attrition model* of psychiatry abolition—which surely does allow for certain types of reform (see Chap. 15)—would that enable you to take a more definitive stand? Or would you still be left with the same unease? On a different but related issue, what balance do you think needs to be struck between emphasizing and de-emphasizing psychiatry?

For the time being, to stick with the issue of what to do if you are on the fence over the question of abolition versus reform, I am aware that allegiances make this issue especially hard for people—for example, who wants to alienate potential allies like comparatively progressive practitioners? What further complicates the matter, there seems to be no models out there on how, when, or under what circumstances to make such a transition. Take the figures in this book, for example. What we mainly see in this book are people who began with little or no foundational critique gaining a compelling critique and consequently substantially shifting their position—while still holding onto reformism. Are there no models out there for a more decisive transition?

Actually, there are several right within this book and seeing what was involved may be helpful to people currently "on the fence". To choose one of these, a shift like this is evident in the dialogue with Breggin. It relates not to a general psychiatry abolition position, but the abolition of one of its "treatments". In this regard, in my exchange with Peter, I observed that he'd become more radical over the years, citing as evidence that he went from finding the push to abolish ECT worrisome to advocating it himself. Whereupon, the dialogue continued as follows:

PB: *It's not exactly more radical…I was very much upfronting freedom as the first value. And that is the basic principle of libertarianism—voluntary relationships. And I came to see that to some degree, that was utopian. It did not take into account the extraordinary abusive influ-*

ences that psychiatrists have on their patients when their patients so-called voluntarily agree to electroshock. What I could see is that hardly any patient ever genuinely agreed to electroshock—I never saw a case where they had a serious discussion with the doctor about the brain-damaging effects.

BB: *Nor are there any cases where they are given honest information.*

PB: *Precisely. So that simply became more apparent to me...The point is that unless someone wanted to kill or badly injure themselves, they would not knowingly submit to electroshock.*

What had happened here? A cutting-edge professional who had always had a profound and totally foundational analysis of what is wrong with electroshock and how inherently damaging it is went from in essence not have an abolitionist position to having one. It is not that he discovered anything new about ECT. It is, rather, that other principles or consider-ations that deterred him from taking an abolitionist position ceased seem-ing so persuasive. One of those principles—and this is one that comes out loud and clear in this exchange—is the libertarian principle of free exchange between equals. Correspondingly, what Peter faced in the courageous way, in which Peter tends to face things, is that this principle in the final analysis is not an adequate one, for, in every exchange, someone has the upper hand—a truth of general relevance but which has special relevance when it comes to psychiatry. How can we speak of equality when one of the play-ers has all the credibility and all the power? When that very same player has the authority to enforce his will? When the other player has the ever-present threat of involuntary incarceration hanging over him?

Before I bring in another consideration that clearly motivated Peter, let me introduce one slightly less clear consideration which may (or may not) have, likewise, played a role. To begin by providing some context: In the 1980s, all of us in the anti-shock movement received incredible help from Peter despite the fact that Peter had not come out in favor of abolishing shock. Now whether or not his reasons were being reported accurately, at the time, a couple of people mentioned to me that Peter was uneasy with others dictating to doctors what they could or could not prescribe—and that this was the reason he was not calling for the abolition of shock.

Fast forward several decades. A few years ago, Peter and three other researchers came together to co-write an article on the electroshocking of children. According to the story told to me, the first author said she wanted them to conclude the article by calling for an investigation into shock—whereupon Peter objected, stating that he was no longer willing

230 EPILOGUE

to be involved in articles calling for investigation—only articles calling for abolition. Herein we see a major turnabout. And how did that turnabout happen? Blatantly, it had nothing to do with making a discovery about ECT for Peter had long had a "damning analysis". If it had to do with the simple reality that other principles that had deterred Peter from coming to this position no longer seemed adequate or perhaps just not as pressing—whether that principle was respecting doctors' right to make their own prescribing decisions or the principle of free and equal exchange. Added to this, he had come to the following conclusions:

1. that no one would knowingly choose to take this "treatment" unless they were intent on harming themselves and
2. psychiatry has shown it cannot be trusted to tell people the truth.

Herein lies a clue as to how you as reader might proceed if you already have a strong foundational critique yourself but are still "on the fence" on whether or not to be abolitionist. To wit: Ask yourself what other principles are entering into your deliberation. Ask yourself if they are adequate. That is, are these principles sound? Or do they need to be modified in some way? Finally, ask yourself what weight to give them in light of the enormity of the harm being done and in light also about what you have come to realize about the profession as a whole. Then, make a balanced judgment on the basis of everything that you know.

Which brings us to several areas of lesser disagreement between the different people in this book but ones nonetheless deserving of thought. And these I likewise invite you to consider. Namely, do you think it is possible to be a professional in this area and *not* inherently be a problem—if only by virtue of your professional status? If so, what do professionals need to keep in mind? If not, how do you see handling the inescapable reality of inequality? How important do you think it is that we de-pathologize our language? Do you think it critical to problematize hegemonic language, even when doing so transparently makes others uncomfortable? If so, why? And if not, why not? And if, like me, you see language as pivotal, how do you see integrating that understanding?

Where do you stand on involving large international organizations like the UN in the fight against psychiatric oppression? Like Peter Breggin, are you worried about the UN gaining power over sovereign states? Or like Tina Minkowitz, are you more concerned about the ability of states to disregard human rights and international law?

To turn to issues over which the vast majority of us who are critical of psychiatry agree, but which, nonetheless, continue to present conundrums: How do you see bringing the left on board? Why do you think that this engagement with the left has been able to happen in Germany with such panache but somehow not in North America? And what is the takeaway lesson here for North American activists?

A few additional questions: How do you see integrating issues of racism, sexism, homophobia, and transphobia more fully? How do you see chipping away at the North-South divide? How do you see protecting movement space? Do you think that the mainstream press is hopeless or do you have ideas on it they might be reached? More generally and most importantly of all, what are your thoughts about how to capture the head, the heart, and the imagination of the general public? For one way or another, with the safeguarding of posterity in the balance, this, we most definitely need to do.

Beyond that, whatever the cause is for which you are struggling, should you find yourself facing seemingly insurmountable obstacles, my invitation is: Do think of the activists in this book. More broadly speaking and on a deeper level still, I hope you will allow the people and the conversations that you have brushed up against in this book to operate at the periphery of your consciousness for they just might be able to be of more help to you than you currently realize. It is not only that you can pick up activist principles that may be transferable or that you may end up so inspired by role models like Julie (see Chap. 13) that you stretch outside of your comfort zone and dare to launch something of monumental importance—though surely that is possible. The point is that there is a degree of commonality to the struggles that we face as beings-in-the-world; moreover, that there is genuine creativity, courage, and wisdom in these stories and narratives. So, if you make space for them in your head and in your heart, like the lingering memory of a long-deceased friend, like a cherished passage from a novel, in the inimical way in which direction happens, they just might illuminate the path on which you tread.

In ending, I thank all the people who have entered into dialogue here, whether as interviewees or readers: Note, such is the state of the world that this reflecting and reimagining that we have been doing is once a dire necessity and a *mitzvah*. Correspondingly, in the spirit of the dedication to Vern Harper with which this book began, in line with the commitment to center Indigeneity, and in acknowledgment of the Indigenous land in which I dwell, let me add *miigwetch*.

APPENDICES

APPENDIX A: LIST OF MOVEMENTS FREQUENTLY REFERENCED AND THE DISTINCTIONS BETWEEN THEM

Name of movement	Distinguishing features
Antipsychiatry	While "way back when", the word "antipsychiatry" referred to anything that critiqued psychiatry or was countering with a different way of understanding and approaching personal problems, now it refers to a social movement which takes the position that psychiatry is fundamentally flawed and harmful, and it works for psychiatry's abolition (e.g., the end of involuntary incarceration and "treatment" and the severing of the relationship between the state and psychiatry). This is not an identity-based movement; anyone can be antipsychiatry just like anyone can be anti-racist; nonetheless, the movement is disproportionately composed of psychiatric survivors. Antipsychiatry folk frequently work with people from the psychiatric survivor movement and the mad movement, including with those who are not actually antipsychiatry, also from the critical psychiatry and the disability rights movement
Critical psychiatry	The critical psychiatry perspective is the perspective of those who want to reform psychiatry as opposed to abolishing it. It is not an identity-based movement though it is a designation and perspective mainly used by progressive or radical "mental health professionals". That said, while they are in the minority, there are some radical professionals who view critical psychiatry as inadequate and so belong, instead, to the antipsychiatry movement

(*continued*)

© The Author(s) 2019
B. Burstow, *The Revolt Against Psychiatry*,
https://doi.org/10.1007/978-3-030-23331-0

234 APPENDICES

(continued)

Name of movement	Distinguishing features
Disability rights movement	The disability rights movement is an anti-oppression movement whose mission is to protect the rights of all people with disabilities and/or would be perceived as having a disability. Most people in the movement have or would be seen as having a disability. This movement theorizes psychiatric survivors as disabled. Nonetheless, there are people in the other movements listed here who would reject the idea that psychiatric survivors are inherently disabled. Most, nonetheless, use the concept at least strategically because it is recognized by the state and can be leveraged in the defense of psychiatric survivor rights
Mad movement	The mad movement is a movement of people who oppose sanism (as to varying degrees *do all the other movements*). This is very much an identity-based movement with the valuing of mad culture particularly emphasized, with it at the same time it being an anti-oppression movement like each of these other movements. Psychiatric survivors form the majority, though allies are also part of it. All of the people in the mad movement are critical of psychiatry. Some are explicitly antipsychiatry, while others are not
Neurodiversity movement	The neurodiversity movement referenced in this book is the *radical* neurodiversity movement only. Participants in this movement take the stand that autism and other divergences from dominant norms of cognition and embodiment are natural manifestations of human neurological diversity rather than "disorders" to be "treated" or eradicated. Correspondingly, the movement itself is mainly identity based
Psychiatric survivor movement	The psychiatric survivor movement is an exclusively identity-based movement of people who have been through the psychiatric system and who challenge it

APPENDIX B: LIST OF COMMONLY USED ABBREVIATIONS

ADHD	Attention Deficit Hyperactivity Disorder
AMA	American Medical Association
APA	American Psychiatric Association
BlPoC	Black and People of Color
CAMH	Centre for Addictions and Mental Health
CAPA	Coalition Against Psychiatric Assault
CRPD	Convention on the Rights of Persons with Disabilities
DSM	*Diagnostic and Statistical Manual of Mental Disorders*
ECT	electroconvulsive therapy
GSK	GlaxoSmithKline

IDA	International Disability Alliance
MIA	Mad in America
NIMH	National Institute of Mental Health
OISE/UT	Ontario Institute for Studies in Education, University of Toronto
SSRI	Selective serotonin reuptake inhibitor
WHO	World Health Organization

APPENDIX C: GLOSSARY OF FREQUENTLY USED TERMS

Colonizing	In this book, while sometimes used literally, generally metaphorically used to refer to a cultural invasion which involves subordinating something to external rule, to the benefit of the external group and/or discipline and to the detriment of what or who is being "colonized". Not to be confused with the literal meaning of "colonizing"
De-professionalize	To take skills or activities out of the domain or the exclusive domain of professionals, such that everyone is engaged in them
Genocide	Refers to the systematic annihilation of an entire people, whether through murder, forbidding of cultural customs, stealing of children, or other means
Hegemonic	Mainstream way of looking at something that has become so accepted that it seems like common sense
Identity politics	Politics based on membership in a specific oppressed group
Medicalizing	Treating something as medical which is not medical
Pathologize	Treat as a disease what is not a disease
Psychiatric survivor	Anyone who has ever been subjected to psychiatry, though often used more restrictively for people who have been incarcerated in a psychiatric facility
Psy/psych disciplines	Interrelated professional disciplines which are part of the helping professions, which are to varying degrees oriented to the psychological, and which to some degree pathologize human beings (e.g., psychiatry, psychology, social work, nursing)
Psychiatrize	Subject people to psychiatry or to the psychiatric system
Sanism	Oppression or inferiorization of people or ways of being hegemonically perceived as psychologically "not normal".

Index

A

Abdillahi, I., 10

Ableism, 91

Abolition, 5, 7, 12, 33, 34, 55, 56, 58, 59, 61, 97, 98, 102, 127, 164, 166, 169, 170, 214, 215, 227–230

Academic freedom, 218

Academic psychiatry, 58, 62–64

Academics/academia, i, 9, 26, 30, 64, 69–81, 111, 112, 116, 119, 127, 169, 209, 216, 218, 219, 227

Activists/activism, i, vi, 1, 2, 4–12, 15–31, 33, 69, 73, 83, 88, 103, 109–119, 121–123, 125–128, 130, 131, 135, 138, 140, 141, 143, 144, 163, 175, 178, 179, 183, 187, 202, 209, 210, 212–216, 218, 223, 225, 226, 231

Aldo Alviani Affair, 210

Alternatives, 7, 9, 10, 43, 96, 98, 105, 118, 123, 130, 164, 204, 207

American Indian Movement (AIM), 16, 28

American Psychiatric Association (APA), 64, 88, 198, 214

Amery, Jean, 22

Anarchism/anarchist, 7–9, 25, 26, 29, 35, 39, 110, 118, 202

Antidepressants, 59, 180, 182, 183, 198

Antipsychiatry, i, vi, 1, 3, 7, 9–12, 15, 35, 49, 51, 55, 56, 61, 69–72, 83–88, 90, 91, 98, 109, 110, 112, 113, 117, 121, 122, 126–128, 135, 139, 141–143, 146, 157, 158, 175, 179, 185, 195, 207, 209–212, 214, 215, 218, 221, 227

See also Psychiatry abolition

Antipsychotics, 36, 152, 154, 198

See also Neuroleptics

Arts, use of, 12, 223

Asylum, 9, 62, 70, 103, 104, 113, 115

Asylum Magazine, 9, 93, 97, 100, 102–104, 191

Attention Deficit Hyperactivity Disorder (ADHD), 47, 63, 65, 184, 198, 199

© The Author(s) 2019
B. Burstow, *The Revolt Against Psychiatry*,
https://doi.org/10.1007/978-3-030-23331-0

238 INDEX

Attrition model of psychiatry
abolition, 12, 214, 215, 228
Autistic, 10, 135–148
See also Neurodivergent
Autogestión Libre-Mente, 109, 110,
112, 118, 119
Autonomous Press, 135, 140

B
Basaglia, Franco, 97, 98, 115
Bauman, Zygmunt, 24
Berlin Runaway House, 9, 83–91, 131
Big Pharma, 64, 227
See also Drug companies;
Pharmaceutical companies
Biological psychiatry, 61, 62, 99,
193, 195
See also Medical model/medical
paradigm
Bonnie Burstow Scholarship in
Antipsychiatry, 218
Breggin, Ginger, 38, 47
Breggin, Peter, 2, 7, 8, 33–49, 102,
197, 214, 225, 228, 230
Buber, Martin, 4
Burstow, Bonnie, i, ii, 1–3, 8, 12, 15,
23, 31, 39, 42, 49, 80, 93, 121,
124, 135, 145, 146, 155, 156,
175, 182, 199, 209–223

C
Capitalism, 24, 26, 28, 29, 37, 91, 116
Castillo, Tatiana, 9, 10, 109–119, 226
Cátedra Libre Franco Basaglia, 109,
111, 114, 119
Center for the Human Rights of Users
and Survivors of Psychiatry, 159
Centre for Addiction and Mental
Health (CAMH), v, vi
Chemical imbalance, 46, 142, 143,
147, 152

Child abuse, 39, 40
Chrisjohn, Roland, 8, 15–31, 96,
194, 226
Clark Institute of Psychiatry, 126
Coalition Against Psychiatric Assault
(CAPA), 85, 158, 175, 178, 179,
188, 212, 215
Cognitive liberty, 10, 135, 138, 144,
147, 148
Cold wet pack, 122–124, 128, 129
College of Physicians and Surgeons of
Ontario (CSPO), 175, 177
Colonialism, 7, 11, 152, 153, 192,
199, 200, 202, 207
Colonization, 11, 16, 24, 27, 154,
155, 192, 195, 199, 202, 203
Community mental health, 98, 115, 196
Compassion, 148
Compulsory normativity, 148
Consumers, 163
Convention on the Rights of Persons
with Disabilities (CRPD), 7, 11,
36, 159–166, 168–171, 173,
222, 225
Cooptation, 62, 101, 114, 153, 154,
166, 171, 184
Counterhegemonic, 3, 12, 227
Counterhegemonic trauma
perspective, 220
Counterhegemonic trauma
practitioners, 12
Creative Empowerment with the
Disenfranchized, 105
Critical discourse analysis, 191
Critical psychiatry, i, 1, 4, 7–9, 51, 53,
55, 56, 93, 100, 102–104, 113

D
Decolonizing Global Mental Health,
193, 207
Democratic psychiatry, 9, 93–106
De-pathologize, 230

INDEX 239

De-professionalization, 44, 106
Diagnostic and Statistical Manual of Mental Disorders (DSM), 61, 94, 139, 163, 196, 198, 199, 220
Diagnostic system, 57, 66
Dialogue, i, ii, 3–6, 8–12, 15–31, 33–49, 51–66, 69–81, 83–91, 93–106, 109–119, 121–132, 135–148, 159–207, 209–223, 225, 227, 228, 231
Direct action/direct activism, vi, 7, 10, 28, 127, 129, 213, 225
Disability, 1, 36, 121, 128, 160–164, 166, 168–171, 173, 174, 191
Disability rights movement, 7, 168, 227
Draining Psychiatry of Respect, 187
Drug companies, 35, 36, 41, 199, 200
See also Big Pharma; Pharmaceutical companies
Dying to please you, 23, 24

E
Electroshock/electroconvulsive therapy, 1, 33, 34, 47, 77, 112, 119, 123, 125, 126, 140, 162, 205, 216, 229
Empathy, 46
Epistemicide, 11, 191–207, 226
Essential Medicines, 184, 198
Eugenics, 38, 155
Experts by experience, 118

F
Fanon, Frantz, 191, 192
Feminism/feminist, 7, 9, 11, 38, 39, 44, 71, 87, 105, 112, 113, 145, 204, 205, 209–211
Feminist therapy, 96
Forced drugging, 123, 147, 161
Forced psychiatric detention, 166

Forced treatment, *see* Involuntary treatment
For Children Being Free of Psychiatric Drugs, 116
Foucault, Michel, 2, 96, 192, 219
Fraud, 22, 35, 36, 76, 181
Free and informed consent, 35, 160–162
Freire, Paulo, 4

G
Gandhi, Mahatma, 195, 202, 213
Genocide, 6–8, 15, 16, 19, 23, 149, 153, 226
GlaxoSmithKline (GSK), 180, 181
Global north, 6, 172, 191, 192, 194, 196, 205
Global south, 6, 163, 171, 172, 194, 203, 205
Gøtzsche, Peter, 35, 60
Grass roots, 111, 127, 131

H
Harper, Vern, v, vi, 231
Healey, David, 2, 180, 182
Hegemony/hegemonic, 1, 21, 23, 167, 170, 204, 219, 230
Hiawatha Asylum for Insane Indians, 155
Holocaust, the, 8, 21–23, 151, 200, 201
Homeless, 43, 83, 84, 89
Horns of a dilemma, 213, 217
Human rights, ii, 2, 10, 11, 37, 40, 78, 79, 128, 140, 159–174, 192, 230

I
Identity politics, 70
Imperialism, 37
Indigenous, v, 6–8, 10, 11, 15–31, 39, 46, 149–158, 194, 226, 227, 231

240 INDEX

Informed consent, 162
Insulin shock, 124, 125
The insurrection of subjected
knowledge, 219
International Classification of Diseases
(ICD), 198
International Conference on Human
Rights and Against Psychiatric
Oppression, 128
International Day of Protest Against
Electroshock, 129
International Disability Alliance
(IDA), 169, 171
International law, 78, 161, 165, 168,
170, 230
International Monetary Fund, 193
Internet, 8, 73, 74, 158, 187
See also Social media
Involuntary treatment, 34, 47, 91,
165, 166, 172
Iroquois, 15, 22, 24, 26, 27, 29
Irrebuttable presumption
of capacity, 160

J
Judges, 36, 164, 165, 181

K
Kuhn, Thomas, 138, 139

L
Laing, R. D., 86
Language, 7, 17, 36, 96, 100, 147,
194, 203, 221, 230
Law suits, 183
Left/left wing, 7, 9, 20, 24, 30, 38,
39, 41, 65, 87, 95, 98, 103, 105,
114, 115, 129, 155, 156,
177–179, 192, 194, 197, 210,
213, 228, 231

Legal capacity, 159, 160, 165, 166
Liberal Mental Health Reform, 99
Libertarian, 7, 34, 35, 38, 229
Libertarianism, 228
Linked services, 197
Lobotomy, 34, 47
Lorde, Audre, 145
Love, 47, 64, 99, 121, 148, 149,
170, 225

M
Mad, 1, 6, 9, 10, 69, 70, 91, 100,
104, 109, 110, 112, 115–117,
119, 135–148
The Mad Farm, 117
Mad for our Rights, 115, 118
Mad In America (MIA), 72, 104, 200
Mad movement, v, 7, 9, 10, 69–71,
87, 100, 109–119, 140, 141,
143, 214, 215, 227
Madness Network News, 71, 72, 123
Mad Pride, 87, 137, 138, 143
Mad studies, 4
Mainstream media, 41, 64, 65
Manual of Rights in Mental Health,
118, 119
Marxism, 7, 8, 26, 105
Medical model/medical paradigm, 10,
122, 131, 138, 185
See also Biological psychiatry
Medication, 16, 29, 47, 59, 65, 152,
160, 185, 189, 192, 196, 197, 221
See also Psychiatric drugs
Mental disorder, 163
Mental health law, 162, 163, 165, 166
Mental Patients Association, 123
Michael, 8, 10, 11, 30, 149–158
Michelle Carter case, 41, 45
Mi'kmaq, 149
Mills, China, 5, 11, 191–207, 226, 227
MindFreedom Hunger Strike, 214
Minkowitz, Tina, 11, 159–174, 225, 230

INDEX 241

Moral management, 99–101
Mosher, Loren, 131
Movement for Global Mental Health, 7, 11, 153, 191–193, 196, 202
Murphy legislation/The Murphy Bill, 73, 78, 184
Mysenburg, Rosie, 181

N
National Institute of Mental Health (NIMH), 62, 131
Neurocosmopolitanism, 135
Neurodivergent, 137, 141, 142, 146, 148
    See also Autistic
Neurodiversity movement, 7, 135, 138, 143, 227
Neurodiversity paradigm, 10, 138, 144
Non-violent resistance, 213

O
Oneida Nation, 15
Ontario Coalition to Stop Electroshock, 126, 212, 216
Opal, 70
Open Dialogue, 62, 101
Oppositional Defiant Disorder, 136, 137
Organizing, 1, 73, 129, 154, 158, 178, 187, 217, 227
The Other Mrs. Smith, 211, 222
Outpatient commitment, 44, 73, 77, 161

P
Paradigm, 1, 7, 129, 138, 139, 143, 145, 147, 148, 161, 167, 213
Paradigm shift, 1, 138, 139, 145, 160, 162, 165, 174
Parents, 1, 2, 5, 10, 11, 16, 22, 42, 79, 81, 85, 136, 149–152, 155, 176, 178, 179, 184–189, 227

Parker, Ian, 9, 93–106, 191
Participatory action research, 75
Pathologize, 197
Paxil, 180, 181
People of color, 7, 77, 156, 211
Pharmaceutical companies, 63, 183, 184
    See also Big Pharma; Drug companies
Phoenix Rising, 72, 121, 127, 210
Pluralism, 11, 203
Popper, Pam, 43, 44
Prefigurative, 1, 110
Presumption of capacity, 11, 160, 162
Prozac, 181, 182
Psychiatric drugging as child abuse, 80
Psychiatric drugs, 1, 11, 21, 26, 40, 42, 43, 46, 47, 59–61, 86, 110, 116, 117, 153, 154, 162, 178, 180, 187, 190, 196, 197, 200, 214
    See also Medication
Psychiatric drug withdrawal, 42
Psychiatric survivor, v, vi, 6, 10, 11, 37, 69, 70, 90, 122–124, 149, 157, 160, 162, 168, 170, 173, 201, 225
Psychiatrization of children/ psychiatrized children/psychiatric assault on children, 39, 186, 190
Psychiatry abolition, 5, 12, 58, 59, 215, 228
    See also Antipsychiatry
Psychiatry and the Business of Madness, 124, 146, 156
Psychology, 16–19, 25, 31, 74, 93–97, 122, 123, 129, 139, 144, 167, 192, 194
Psychotherapy, 94
PsychOut, 69, 130, 217
Psy disciplines/psy professions, 8, 16, 18, 94, 95, 167, 197, 207
PTSD, 18, 23, 144, 145
Public hearings, 158

242　INDEX

Q

Queen St. Mental Health Centre, 122, 209, 215

Queer, 135–138, 140, 141, 146

R

Racism, v, 1, 7, 8, 15–31, 76, 77, 91, 156, 194, 200, 205, 231

Radical Feminist Therapy, 15

Rappaport study, 59

Reclaiming words, 70, 100, 103

Reform, 7, 9, 49, 55, 56, 61–63, 65, 98, 102–104, 114, 165, 166, 227, 228

Reporters, 51, 53–55, 64, 65, 129, 178, 180

Reserves/reservations, 6, 16, 21, 23, 26, 85, 151, 153

Revolution, 62, 99, 117, 159

Rights, ii, 2, 7, 10–12, 17, 18, 37, 39–41, 47, 52, 53, 55–57, 61, 78, 79, 96, 118, 119, 128, 140, 159–174, 192, 211, 228, 230

Royal Commission Report on Indigenous People, 21

S

Sane literate, 222

Sanism, v, 10, 86

Santos, De Sousa, 204

Schizoaffective disorder, 176

Schizophrenia, 55, 57, 70, 131, 211

Schwarz, Alan, 65

Seclusion, 129

Selective serotonin reuptake inhibitors (SSRIs), 182

Self-help, 91, 95, 115, 131

Sexism, 1, 91, 205, 231

Simpson's Paradox, 18

Sit-in, 126, 212

The Sixties Scoop, 10, 149, 150, 153

Small movement organizations, 212

Social media, 41, 42, 65, 72–74, 76, 138, 140, 183

See also Internet

Social model of disability, 162, 173

Solidarity, 118, 147, 148, 169

Soteria House, 131

SSRI stories, 181

Stealing of children, 151

Stimulants, 176, 177, 184

Stop Shocking Our Mothers and Grandmothers, 112

Strategic activism, 12, 213, 214, 223

Strategic resistance, 105, 106

Study 329, 180, 181

Suicide, 6, 8, 16, 21, 23, 152, 154, 176, 182

Surviving Race, 76

Survivor movement, 11, 37, 45, 71, 83, 113, 128, 166, 171, 205

Szasz, Thomas, 1, 2, 5, 17, 18, 30, 34, 97, 98, 123, 180

T

Teachable moments, 218

Teachers, 2, 81, 117, 135, 185, 186, 198, 222

Teaching as activism, 7

Telling of our stories, 157

Tenney, Lauren, 5–7, 9, 69–81, 188, 226, 227

Torture, 36, 123, 161

Trans/transgendered people, 6, 85

Trauma, 12, 136, 140, 144, 145, 151, 152, 220, 223

Truth and Reconciliation, 22

Two-spirit/two spirited, 152, 154

U

United Nations (UN), 2, 36, 37, 40, 128, 140, 162, 164, 165, 168, 170, 171, 174, 230
UN rapporteurs on torture, 36
Users, 102, 110, 115, 118, 119, 159, 166, 168, 171, 172, 191, 195, 205

V

Varga, Oriel, 209
(de)Voiced, 74

W

Walker, Nick, 10, 135–148, 225
Weinberg, Michael, 214

Weitz, Don, 5, 8, 10, 121–132, 211, 216, 225, 227
Whitaker, Robert, 1, 2, 5, 7, 8, 36, 51–66, 184, 222
Wichera, Kim, 9, 83–91
Wittgenstein, Ludwig, 8, 17–19, 30
Wood, John David, 175–177, 179, 184, 188
Wood, Julie, 7, 11, 175–190, 225
World Bank, 193
World Health Organization WHO), 36, 37, 55, 163, 164, 184, 193, 198
World Network of Users and Survivors of Psychiatry (WNUSP), 159, 168, 169

GPSR Compliance
The European Union's (EU) General Product Safety Regulation (GPSR) is a set of rules that requires consumer products to be safe and our obligations to ensure this.

If you have any concerns about our products, you can contact us on

ProductSafety@springernature.com

In case Publisher is established outside the EU, the EU authorized representative is:

Springer Nature Customer Service Center GmbH
Europaplatz 3
69115 Heidelberg, Germany

www.ingramcontent.com/pod-product-compliance
Lightning Source LLC
Chambersburg PA
CBHW071233200425
25427CB00004B/37